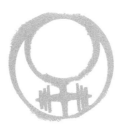

*LIFT LIKE A GIRL*

Be More, Not Less.

ISBN    978-1-61961-844-2   Paperback

       978-1-61961-843-5   Ebook

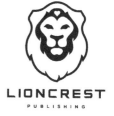

# LIFT LIKE A GIRL

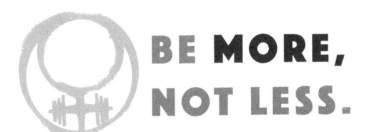 **BE MORE, NOT LESS.**

## NIA SHANKS

*To Kristy, Mom, and Meliah*

Here's to strong women.

May we know them.

May we be them.

May we raise them.

—*Unknown*

# CONTENTS

# FOREWORD

*Lift Like a Girl* is not only about the power of resistance training to transform the female physique; it's a completely new way of thinking about food and fitness. As you read this book, you'll discover how lifting weights combined with a sensible eating plan and a handful of changes in mindset will transform not only your body, but also your whole life and the way you feel about yourself every day.

Woven throughout Nia's advice on training, nutrition, and mindset are the central themes of simplicity, flexibility, and sustainability. These are three of the most important keys to success, but they are sorely lacking in most mainstream fitness, diet, and weight loss programs.

The mindset strategies in *Lift Like a Girl* are not limited to setting goals or thinking positive—they are dramatic paradigm shifts in how you look at food, exercise, and your own body. It's virtually the opposite of how most dieters think, and even the opposite of what many fitness experts tell you. These ideas may challenge your current views, but if you're open-minded and willing to rethink what you believe in a few vital areas, these strategies could change your life.

Once you've digested the lessons from this book, you'll understand the pitfalls of focusing only on appearance or weight, especially if your goals are influenced by other people's standards. You're likely to agree with Nia that happiness is not achieved by reaching a certain measurement or bodyweight.

Yes, you can pursue the aesthetic changes you want, but thinking beyond appearance or a number on the scale will help you achieve and appreciate improvements in your health, strength, fitness, and confidence as well. You'll also realize that when you pursue the right type of fitness goals with the right mindset, much of the joy is in the journey.

You'll learn what it means to shift your mindset to focus on "more, not less" and learn to recognize the dangers of all-or-nothing attitudes. You'll see why the extreme restrictions and rules of conventional weight loss programs are unnecessary and usually backfire. You'll understand how allowing more flexibility, being less rigid, and eating foods you enjoy is possible and gets you better results in the long run.

Nia's nutrition plan is not a fad; it's not even a diet—it's a handful of simple habits to adopt every day that become your new lifestyle. You can eat foods you like, and you'll find no lists of forbidden or evil foods. In fact, you'll learn why it's not productive to dichotomize foods into good and bad. The plan is not complicated either—it's so simple, you might wonder how it works so well. The answer is that a small number of important fundamentals give you almost all of your results. Focus on those vital few, and you don't need to stress over the many trivial details.

The training plan is also remarkably simple. You might even be tempted to do more, but *Lift Like a Girl* explains how working hard on a handful of highly effective exercises and following proven principles of progressive training gives you incredible bang for your buck without spending hours in the gym.

The training program is not about extreme workouts that pummel you to exhaustion, but training that makes you feel good and that you actually enjoy. You'll avoid vicious cycles of exercising for punishment or guilt and learn self-compassion. You'll train with purpose and include performance, function, health, and strength in your goals.

In the past, many women shied away from the weight room, but today we're entering a fantastic new era in the fitness world where more and more women appreciate the benefits of serious strength training. Nia is leading this movement by example; she is one strong woman. She has also been through and overcome all the same dieting and body image challenges that many women struggle with, so you'd be hard-pressed to find a better coach and a better book to show you how you can do it too.

Tom Venuto, author of
*Burn the Fat, Feed the Muscle*

# DISCLAIMER

This book is for educational and entertainment purposes and should not be used as a substitute for professional medical treatment, advice, or diagnosis. Consult your physician or health-care provider before changing your diet or starting a strength training program to determine if it is right for your needs.

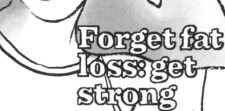

DECEMBER 2017

# Lift Like a Girl

## How to feel awesome

## Forget fat loss: get strong

# BE MORE, NOT LESS

# INTRODUCTION
# The Ugly Side of Health and Fitness

The health and fitness industry has done a fantastic job of making women dislike their bodies, and themselves.

Browse the health section at your local bookstore, scroll through social media feeds of fitness professionals, glance at fitness magazines in the checkout aisle of the grocery store. It's abundantly clear what modern health and fitness is about: losing fat, getting into a smaller clothing size, fixing flaws, and building "perfect" body parts. Physical endowments like a defined midsection and sculpted butt are highlighted, while tips to reduce cellulite and the newest fat-scorching workout are plastered on magazine covers and littered across social media.

You can finally love your body and be happy once you attain these goals, or so we're led to believe. Happiness, it seems, is just a couple of smaller pant sizes or one perfectly sculpted body part away.

Look around much of the health and fitness world, and the underlying themes become abundantly clear. The effectiveness of a workout is determined by how exhausted you were at the end or how sore you felt the next day. And when it comes to food, you need to be on a rigid, restrictive diet, and you must follow it perfectly, without deviation.

Behind these messages is a fundamental principle that saturates the health and fitness industry: your priority, as a woman, is to build a leaner, more attractive body free from flaws, at any cost necessary. Once you achieve a goal, it's time to move on to the next thing on your body that you can improve.

Is it any wonder so many women dislike not just their bodies, but themselves?

What it means to be a woman, according to the health and fitness industry:

- Constantly dieting is just part of being a woman.
- You can attain happiness by reaching a smaller number on the bathroom scale.
- It's normal to spend extra time working out either to atone for the "food sins" you committed yesterday or to get ahead of the ones you'll commit tomorrow.
- Depriving yourself of your favorite foods means you're "disciplined."
- If you don't finish a workout exhausted or sore the next day, you didn't work hard enough.
- How you look (still) matters most.

Health and fitness has been relegated to the lowest possible denominator: the superficial has replaced the substantive.

"Health" and "fitness" nowadays really aren't so much about health or fitness as they are about achieving superficial standards, at any cost necessary, and with a blatant disregard for other more important components of what truly defines health and fitness.

In other words, it's not about how healthy or fit you are; it's about how healthy and fit you look.

The superficial focus has ushered in obsessive eating habits, negative self-image, frustration, guilt, dissatisfaction, determining self-worth by numbers (e.g., the scale, pant size, etc.), and a surplus of costly gimmicks and worthless supplements.

And it's nonsense. Actually, that word isn't nearly strong enough. It is flagrant bullshit.

Society is quick to label features of a woman's body as flaws, and then offer to sell us the solution. One common example: cellulite. We've been conditioned to see it on ourselves and respond with disgust. "Cellulite is bad," we've been led to believe; it's a flaw we must fix. After all, if it weren't, surely there wouldn't be dozens of creams and treatments to make it go away.

Cellulite is not a flaw. It *is* a natural, common feature that approximately 90 percent of women have. While it can be reduced through proper nutrition and exercise, it's still *not* a flaw. People are quick to point it out in disgust because it's visible fat, and fat is a word women have been taught to loathe and fear.

But that's stupid. We all have fat, and we need it to be healthy and vibrant. We need to remove the emotional response tied to that word. For example, "I have cellulite on the back of my legs. That's bad, so it makes me less attractive."

To reiterate, cellulite is not a flaw. It's as common as gray hair, wrinkles, crow's feet, stretch marks, and other signs of living life. And we need to stop labeling them as such and choose to put our energy and attention toward positive, rewarding, empowering actions.

Health and fitness is a multibillion-dollar industry—per year. It will incessantly poke your insecurities and gladly create new ones just to sell you a "solution." Intelligent marketers know how impatient humans are, and they're happy to play to our innate desire for instant gratification. They point out a "flaw" (You have unsightly cellulite!) that makes us self-conscious and present us with tantalizing products and programs that promise to deliver quick results (You can be more beautiful within a short time with our revolutionary product.). They know which buttons to push so we reach right over our common sense to whip out the credit card if we believe their solution just might work.

This brings up another problem with fad diets, fitness programs, and "hacks" that promise drastic results in a few short weeks. We're told if we "go all in" and do the program or diet perfectly, we'll achieve results that provide overwhelming happiness. Not only is "perfectly" following such a thing an extreme challenge, but we never stop and ask, "What will I do once this is over?"

Most diets and programs come to an end. What are you supposed to do when it's over? (Besides sign up for the next one.)

Instead of yet another extreme, strict regimen, why not try something different? Something that truly works so you not only achieve great results, but you can *maintain* them without a tremendous amount of effort—and you can do it for the rest of your life.

Uncomfortable truth: a drastically different-looking body is not attainable with only a few weeks of hard work. This is marketing BS designed to make the sale, not to help you sustainably achieve your goals. To maintain the results you achieved this month well into next year, it's crucial to develop sustainable habits you actually enjoy.

If you want to feel confident in your favorite pair of jeans or swimsuit, this book will get you there. But I want to make sure that, come next year, you don't find yourself saying, "I gained a bunch of weight. Help me get my body back." I love training people, but I do not love helping people get their bodies "back" year in and year out. Rather, my goal is to help you develop a sustainable lifestyle so you can maintain the results you achieve into the next year, and the year after.

That's only possible if you enjoy the process (at least most of the time) and it fits into your life (instead of dominating it).

The way you eat and work out should enhance, and *fit into*, your life. It shouldn't dominate or consume it.

If you hate the process or feel like your life must revolve around it, you know you won't keep doing it.

## THE RESET

I have a challenge for you as you dive into this book. Disregard everything you've been told about nutrition and working out, and definitely the nonsense perpetuating the notion that self-worth fluctuates with the number on the scale, or your ability to sculpt perfect body parts.

1. **FORGET WHAT YOU'VE BEEN TOLD ABOUT EXERCISE AND STRENGTH TRAINING.**

   The effectiveness of a workout is not determined by how fatigued you are at the end of it, or how sore you are the following day.

2. **FORGET WHAT YOU'VE BEEN TOLD ABOUT NUTRITION.**

   You don't have to avoid any foods or entire food groups (unless told otherwise by a doctor, of course), or follow obsessive guidelines.

3. **FORGET WHAT YOU'VE BEEN TOLD MATTERS MOST FOR TRACKING YOUR PROGRESS.**

   Success is not measured by how much you deprive yourself of certain foods, and you don't have to reach a certain bodyweight or clothing size to be happy and appreciate your body.

Despite what's plastered on headlines and magazines, health and fitness should not be defined by a physical image. It should be defined by how you feel in your own skin and the way you view food and moving your body. It should be about building a lifestyle rooted in sustainable habits.

In an industry that tries to sell all things *less* (weigh less, eat less, etc.) as the path to happiness, it's time to choose a life of *more*.

Let me be clear about what I'm *not* saying here. There's nothing wrong with having a defined midsection or thigh gap or back dimples or any other physical feature. Many women have those traits, and that's awesome. Many women don't have those traits, and that's awesome. *No physical feature makes a body objectively inferior or superior*. The problem isn't having those features—it's when physical features or an "ideal image" are an obsessive, consuming desire or determinant of self-worth and take precedence over physical and mental health. Shredded abs aren't valuable if the lifestyle required to achieve and maintain them is wrought with misery.

Likewise, I'm not suggesting that weight loss that leads to lower blood pressure and joints that no longer ache is bad. Losing inches off your waist or thighs is not bad because, after all, it's your body. You're entitled to do what you want with it. What makes chasing *less* a problem is when we think those smaller numbers in and of themselves will make us happy. That we *must* reach those standards to increase our self-worth or beauty. There's a huge difference between wanting to lose weight and transform your body because you despise how you look and thinking that doing so will finally make you happy and increase your self-worth, and losing weight to improve your health (or because it's a side effect from eating well and getting stronger in the gym) and thinking that doing so makes you a better version of yourself, *apart from* the physical changes.

Choosing to be *more* instead of chasing less requires a mindset shift, but the payoff is monumental. It means discovering and embracing methods that make you feel fantastic, powerful, and confident. It means becoming *more* of who you are, and who you want to be.

> Be *more*. Strive to do more of the things that make you feel great, strong, confident, empowered, healthy, and alive. Avoid (or at least minimize) all things *less* that do the opposite.

That mindset is accompanied by an intense focus on function, strength, longevity, and health. Everything else—losing fat, or getting a toned look that comes from proper strength training and nutrition—will simply be *side effects*. If reaching a bodyweight squat in your workouts combined with consistently practicing simple nutrition guidelines means you also drop several pounds of fat in the process, so be it. The real difference will be in the mindset that led to those changes. It may be hard to imagine now, but it truly is possible to experience those changes without being obsessed with dropping fat. It happens when you're chasing *more*—in the form of adding weight to the barbell and eating more of the foods that give you energy, make you feel great, and improve overall health.

This journey you're about to embark on will make you feel awesome, an element often missing from many fad programs and diets. It's about gaining strength that makes your life easier, less stressful, and more enjoyable. It's about eating well, not just for the goal of looking better, but to nourish yourself so you can grow stronger and more resilient. It's about building a body that serves you and allows you to live your life to the fullest.

It's about creating a sustainable *lifestyle*. All the things you do for your health—strength training, eating well, harnessing an empowered mindset—become things you do because they're part of who you are.

## A TRIP TO THE DARK SIDE OF HEALTH AND FITNESS

I had the privilege of being raised in a healthy household. My mom was an aerobics instructor in the 1980s and later became the first woman personal trainer in our area. My dad was an avid runner and coached many of my youth sports teams. Eating well and being active was just something we did—it was never a challenge for me.

When I was thirteen, I was in a car accident that left me with a broken growth plate in my right ankle, along with other injuries. Months later, when the cast was removed, my physical therapy took place at my mom's gym. During rehab sessions I'd catch a glimpse of her training clients. Once therapy concluded and I continued to regain the strength and muscle I'd lost, my mom introduced me to strength training. I loved it from day one.

By the time I was sixteen, I was consistently strength training, as well as "training" my friends for fun throughout high school. By nineteen, I became a certified personal trainer and later acquired a bachelor of science in exercise physiology from the University of Louisville.

When I became a certified trainer at nineteen, I spent more and more time at the gym. As a result, I heard numerous conversations about diet and nutrition. I'd hear young women my age bemoaning their meals that week. It wasn't just, "Oh my God. I can't believe I ate this." They knew the exact calorie counts for every bite that went into their mouths. "You had a cheeseburger and fries? Here's how many calories you ate..."

These conversations made me curious. I knew how to eat well, how to lose fat and build muscle, but I had never personally tracked how many calories I ate each day. The more I heard people talking about how many calories they consumed and the latest diet they were on, the more I felt obligated to experiment. After all, if a client asked about a certain diet, I wanted to have a knowledgeable opinion. I experimented with what I learned—counting macronutrients (grams of fat, carbohydrates, and protein) and eating the "perfect" combination of fat, protein, and carbs.

And when the clean food/dirty food dichotomy flooded the fitness scene, I immediately adopted the philosophy as my way of life. After all, I was a young trainer who was still completing her education. If I was going to inspire and motivate people, I felt that I needed to look phenomenal. I was already lean and toned, but I figured I could always be leaner and even more toned.

The problem wasn't the goal itself; the problem was my mentality around it. Even though I was trying to get more toned and lean, I was doing it to fulfill what I believed others expected of me. I was extremely strict with my diet, to the point where it negatively affected my social life. My life was dominated by how I ate and when I worked out. I tried to convince myself that the more body fat I dropped, the happier and more valuable I would be, and the more credibility I'd receive from fellow trainers and potential clients.

It was innocent enough, at first. But without noticing, what began as self-education and experimentation gradually became extreme, compulsive restriction.

Not only was I meticulously tracking calories (including a stick of gum), but I was also religiously avoiding any and all dirty food. This included desserts, candy (even a tiny piece was off-limits), processed meats like hot dogs and sausage, and even butter (too many calories). I was so obsessed with eating "clean" that if I made plans to go out to eat, I'd find the menu online and study it before we left to find the cleanest and lowest-calorie option. (And you'd better believe I made sure the waiter heard me when I said, "No butter on anything.")

My life was tallied up in lean protein, whole grains, eggs, steamed vegetables, fruit, and low-fat dairy. If a cookie showed up on my horizon, I'd mentally slap it to the ground. Ice cream? Pizza? A bite of dessert? You're nuts. I'm a serious trainer. Food for me, at that time, was just fuel. To have it be anything more meant I was undisciplined.

I prided myself on my discipline to eat "clean" and train hard. I never missed a workout, never ate "bad" foods. But one night, I had an experience that would drastically affect my life for the next several years.

I returned home after going out to eat with my family; I ate a typical meal of salmon, steamed veggies (you heard me say no butter, right?), and salad (dressing on the side). While that meal satisfied my physical hunger, my taste buds felt neglected and in need of satisfaction. "I've been good for so long," I thought proudly and wistfully as I drifted into the pantry and started snacking on whatever I found that sounded good. Without realizing it, I made my way from there to the refrigerator and, same thing, grabbed various foods and started mindlessly munching away.

It's difficult to describe what happened. It was like I went into a trance. I just kept eating and eating. And eating.

About half an hour lapsed before the feeding frenzy came to a halt. I came to my senses and realized my stomach was stuffed. Not stuffed like I just ate a big Thanksgiving meal, but stuffed to the point of feeling nauseated. I couldn't lie on my back because I was so full that it was hard to breathe. It dawned on me that I had just inhaled a massive quantity of food. And not just any food, but dirty food: pretzels, cheese, crackers, large spoonfuls of peanut butter, even cookies. I was horrified by the way my brain blanked out—where had the time gone? Accompanying that fear was guilt from having eaten all the "forbidden" foods I had successfully avoided for months, and so much of them. How did I lose control like that?

At the time, I was naïve enough to believe that was a one-time episode. But it was the first of hundreds of binges I'd experience over the next several years. It was a catalyst to growing self-hatred, which led me to experiment with numerous diets, hoping they would help me break free from the compulsive habits I'd developed, and the fat that piled on as a result.

The bingeing episodes grew in frequency and quantity. But I couldn't stop. I felt powerless. In desperation, I tried to restrict the amount of food I would eat at mealtimes to undo the damage, and to prepare for the inevitable binge in the near future.

One particular binge I recall with clarity: I devoured an entire jar of peanut butter, a whole box of cereal, and half a loaf of bread. And this was less than an hour after I ate a "clean" breakfast of scrambled eggs and sautéed veggies. I can still feel the discomfort in my stomach and, right beside it, the immense disgust and shame I felt for my lack of self-control.

The mirrors at home and in the gym offered a constant reminder of how the binge eating was changing my body against my will: my clothes were becoming too small, my muscle definition faded away, my face became a shape I no longer recognized, and stretch marks appeared on my butt and thighs. I wanted to scream at this alien figure looking back at me. She made me feel like a fraud, a failure. I was a trainer, but who would take me seriously when I looked this way?

Since I couldn't make myself stop binge eating, I turned to the one thing I could control: exercise. I began to exercise harder, and for longer periods of time, as frequently as possible. The morning after a binge, I'd wake up early and hit the cardio machines for at least half an hour before my first client showed up. Between clients I would lift, do more cardio, cramming in as much exercise as I could. Then I'd go home and run a dozen hill sprints. To compound this punishment for the previous binge, I'd add in extra calorie restrictions to prepare for the binge that would inevitably follow.

The frequent, high-intensity exercise turned something I once loved—strength training—into a loathsome chore. Into punishment. Into something I did because I hated my body and wanted desperately to change how it looked. All other physical activity was merely a means to burn calories; moving my body and even hobbies were no longer enjoyable or things that made me feel good.

It was a grueling cycle: binge, extreme guilt and shame, desperately try to restrict my food intake, work out as hard and as often as possible, more bingeing, more guilt and shame.

My stomach was distended in near-constant pain, but as soon as the pain dissipated, I'd eat again. My intestines and stomach felt like they were on the brink of explosion. Finally, I visited the doctor to get a checkup, though I conveniently neglected to tell her about my binge eating habit. (Do *not* do this. If you have a problem or concern, tell your doctor so he/she can help you. I have a wonderful doctor and did her a disservice by withholding information.) I told her my stomach was swelling and was in constant pain. She ordered a round of tests, and it exposed part of the problem: my gallbladder was leaking into my

If you're battling disordered eating habits or an eating disorder, one of the best steps you can take is to seek help from a qualified professional. These resources may be a good place to start: *www.nationaleatingdisorders. org, www.eatingdisorderhope. com,* and *bedaonline.com.*

stomach, which contributed to the pain and swelling.

This daily cycle of bingeing/exercising/restricting my food as much as possible went on for more than three years. More than three years of punishing myself with intense, frequent workouts. More than three years of food dominating my thoughts every waking moment. More than three years of hating my body and the person I had become. More than three years of thinking I would finally be happy once I got my old body back and desperately trying anything that promised fast results (but these only exacerbated the binge eating). More than three years of wondering if I was going to have to struggle with this issue for the rest of my life.

I thought my self-hate was fuel and motivation that would help transform my body into something that would finally make me happy. I didn't realize then that you cannot "hate your way" to happiness.

The point in sharing this story with you is to let you know that I've experienced how terrifying, and infuriating, it can be to feel out of control of your body. To be on a never-ending journey of *less*, where I'm trying to eat less every day, trying to weigh less, trying to shrink down to a smaller jean size, trying to whittle away parts of my body I'd glare at with disgust. I was consumed by trying to be *less* because I thought doing so would finally allow me to love my body, to feel worthy and beautiful.

If parts of that experience are similar to your own, please know it's not just you who is going through it. Sadly, it's common, but it's not something everyone is willing to discuss openly. You're not alone. You're not broken. There is a way out.

And if you bought this book to begin (or to simplify) your health and fitness lifestyle or to get strong and become awesome, and you can't relate to my personal experience—great. I don't want you to know what it's like to hate your body. If you love your body now, this book is going to help you love it even more.

Rest assured, no matter what your health and fitness journey has looked like or what you want to achieve with it, *Lift Like a Girl* will get you there. Simple, flexible, and empowering, the programs in this book are designed to ensure that women like you can live your life around all things *more*.

## WHAT DOES IT MEAN TO LIFT LIKE A GIRL?

Growing up, you likely heard what was meant to be a condescending phrase, "You hit like a girl!" or "You throw like a girl!" Boys, and even men, are still told they do something "like a girl" when other guys are trying to insult them.

The intended message is clear: Doing something "like a girl" means being inferior, worse, less than.

This book annihilates that condescension. Far from being less than, lifting *like a girl* is empowering, intelligent, purposeful, and awesome. It's not just about lifting more weight and getting stronger (though that is a part of it). It's about becoming *more* in every sense.

*Lift Like a Girl* is shorthand for an empowered, sustainable, lifestyle approach to health and fitness. It's all about choosing to use how you eat and move your body as a way to feel great about yourself. It's something that will enhance your life, not dominate it. It will ultimately reduce your stress, not add to it.

*Lift Like a Girl* starts with deciding what matters to *you*, as we'll explore in the next chapter. It puts you in charge of setting your goals and choosing your values. You don't have to passively absorb what society says you're supposed to look like or what you're supposed to do. You don't have to hang your happiness on some specific outcome like a number on a scale or a clothing size. Instead, you get to wake up feeling great about yourself. Because guess what? You're entitled to feel great about yourself.

*Lift Like a Girl* means measuring success by how you feel, how you perform in your workouts, the habits you practice and build, your health (e.g., blood pressure, blood lipid profile, etc.), and a willingness to discover the incredible things your body can do.

*Lift Like a Girl* means building a stronger, healthier body that enhances your everyday life in ways you may not expect. I know it sounds like a tall order, but getting stronger and eating well can make the rest of your life better. You don't have to take my word for it—you'll see some incredible experiences from other women in this book. Best of all, you'll experience it for yourself when you put the information into practice.

## LIFT LIKE A GIRL IN REAL LIFE

"A smallish dead tree fell, blocking my drive. I was able to roll it out of the way BY MYSELF and proceed to work. I couldn't have done it three months ago. Thanks, Nia! BTW, I'm fifty-one. Larger trees are poised to fall. I say, 'Bring 'em on!'"

*Lift Like a Girl* means choosing to value things by their ultimate function. Physical strength is functional. Forging the right mindset is functional. Building a healthy body is functional. A sculpted midsection, while you may love how it looks, is not functional. Functional results are what can influence happiness, because of what they allow you to do, be, and achieve. The aesthetic changes they deliver (e.g., slim midsection) are side effects.

This book provides the necessary tools for feeling confident and becoming more. I happen to think they're the best tools, and not only because they've made a significant difference in my life. I've worked with countless women, in person and through online coaching programs, who have reported that the simple strength training and nutrition guidelines in this book have revolutionized the way they live. You'll read some of their stories, and how the outcome of these tools is as diverse as the women who use them.

I'm tired of seeing strong, spectacular women feeling as if they're not enough because they don't see a certain number on the scale or have a specific body shape. It's time to demand more. I want you to experience the relief and freedom from shedding those constricting demands. I want you to be excited at the prospect of doing something that makes you feel good. I want you to discover the incredible things your body can do instead of obsessing over the way you look and whether it matches some external standard you were convinced was important. I want you to look in the mirror and see a body that serves you, and then leave the mirror and go out and live your real life, more awesome than ever.

I want you to shatter the mold that women have been encouraged to cram themselves into, and actively choose for yourself what *you* want and what's important to *you*.

If you've had a similar experience to mine, where you spent long periods of time obsessing over food and disliking parts of your body and working out for the sole goal of transforming your body because you thought doing so would make you happy, then all this may seem impossible. I know you could feel a tendency, once you read the guidelines and workouts in this book, to feel as if you have to do extra to achieve noticeable results. (Especially when you see how simple this program is.)

Let me take you on this journey, and I will show you how simple and enjoyable strength training, nutrition, and harnessing the right mindset can be. It's a journey completely free of obsession, guilt, demands of perfection, and exhaustion. As you take these first few steps, you'll find a whole new way to experience health and fitness. It doesn't feel like punishment. It doesn't feel like checking off a box on your to-do list each day, or gauging your self-worth based on how "good" you were in the kitchen. It's not defined by rigidity and restriction and deprivation.

It can, and will, be something you look forward to and enjoy doing.

It's been a privilege to work with spectacular women from all walks of life: moms, grandmothers, business owners, doctors, farmers, and teachers. Sadly, many were unaware of how spectacular they were. Society has ingrained in us that how we look matters more than anything else, and I've seen how it can hold women back—and I've experienced it myself. But once they start strength training with the goal of getting stronger instead of burning calories, and eating for health and performance instead of obsessing over fat loss, everything changes—first in their minds, and then in their bodies. There's nothing more powerful than a woman realizing she is more than the number on a scale or the size of her pants. She discovers that she is stronger than she ever knew she could be, and she loves how it feels. The confidence built inside the gym helps her soar through her life outside the gym. That is what *Lift Like a Girl* is about.

## NEW LIFESTYLE, NEW LANGUAGE

You may embrace new words and mantras as you read this book. Don't be surprised when you find yourself saying:

*I'm training to get strong.*

*I'm going to eat more of the things that make me feel great.*

*I'm not trying to make the number on the scale go down; the goal is to make the weight on the barbell go up.*

*I'm proud of what my body can do, and not just for how it looks.*

*I eat my favorite foods on occasion with absolutely no guilt.*

*I work out because it makes me feel great and improves my overall life, not because I need to burn off the cookies I ate last night.*

*I feel confident, I have energy, I'm getting stronger, and I'm healthy; it doesn't matter what the scale says.*

*I am capable of more than I realized: physically and mentally.*

These are only a few examples, and you'll no doubt add your own to the list, but as you can see, health and fitness—done the *Lift Like a Girl* way—is about empowerment and, ultimately, becoming the version of yourself that makes you feel the most awesome.

If you're used to typical fad diets that are rigid and strict, or working out solely for a huge calorie burn, this concept may seem foreign. And I think that's a good thing. It means you already tried all the other methods. It's time to try something different. Something better.

There's a health and fitness paradox, and you've probably experienced it: The more you want to lose weight and look better, the harder that goal seems to achieve. My point is this: How many diets and workout programs have you tried hoping it would be "the one"? Why not, instead, try to strive for something that could provide greater rewards?

Become stronger, more capable, confident, and awesome. Make better health an important goal (e.g., improved blood pressure, cholesterol, triglycerides, etc.). Strive to be emotionally healthy and mentally strong. Develop simple habits that will serve you for a lifetime. Embrace the challenge of learning new exercises and, if necessary, getting out of your comfort zone (because this is an opportunity to grow and, at the risk of being annoyingly redundant, be more). Choose something functional, and allow the positive physical changes to be by-products of your newfound, ever-growing awesomeness. Something that can improve you as a human. Something deeper than a superficial badge of honor.

> " The truth will set you free, but first it will piss you off.
> —Gloria Steinem

We're still sold the idea that our physical appearance is the most important thing about us. That should piss us off. Only then can we choose to be strong and bold. Only then can we refuse to be demoted to an ornament or decoration.

Our minds have been polluted with images and messages about "what a real woman" is and how we should eat and what we should do with our bodies. These messages cloud our vision and distort our perceptions. We no longer look at food as just food—we see potential fat gain, or loss. We don't look at physical activity as something that makes us feel great—we tally success by calories burned and fatigue accumulated.

We don't see an innocent number on the scale or in the tag of our jeans; we see numbers that have come to define us and determine our value. Moving our bodies and choosing our meals becomes more about punishment, fixing flaws, and burning calories instead of doing things that make us *feel good*.

Even if you live to see your 107th birthday, your life will still be too short and precious to justify hating parts of your body and revolving your life around a rigid, miserable diet and workouts that leave you exhausted and discouraged because you were chasing an image someone else said you should have. That time is best spent building a stronger, healthier, more resilient mind and body so you can thrive and enjoy to the greatest extent possible your short time on this planet.

The body you have now is the only one you're going to get— you can't trade it in for a different model. The only true option (filled with freedom, I might add) is to take care of that body and make the most of it. Take the time to discover what makes it strong and unique. This is exactly what you'll do with the *Lift Like a Girl* strength training programs.

You're about to begin an exciting, rewarding journey that will allow you to discover your body in an entirely new way. Let's get started.

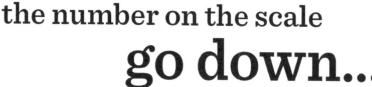

Forget about making
the number on the scale
# go down...

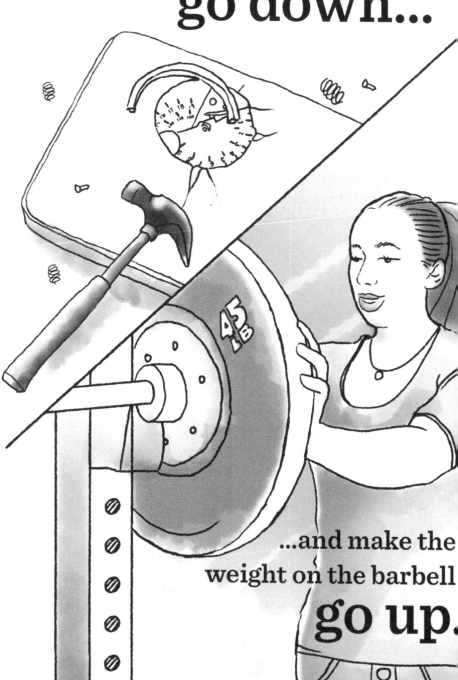

...and make the
weight on the barbell
## go up.

# CHAPTER I

# Strength Training for Your Mind

Imagine you're on a beautiful beach. The sky is cloudless. The sand is powder soft, and the water is the perfect temperature.

Now imagine what you're doing on this picturesque beach. Jumping in the waves? Practicing your hang-ten? Running with your dog? Building sand castles with your kids? Walking along the shore picking up seashell souvenirs? Whatever you're doing, you're having fun, enjoying the feel of sun and water on your skin and the energy pulsing through your body. Hours slip by unnoticed.

Imagine how you feel when you get home that day. Tired, sure, but in the best way possible. Your body's worn out, but you're still high on endorphins. You're ravenous, and anything you eat will taste delicious. After a good meal you plan to get cozy on the couch in your pajamas, knowing you'll drift to sleep in a matter of minutes.

When was the last time exercise felt this good?

# RETHINKING WHAT'S "NORMAL"

The word *exercise* was probably the last thing on your mind while you were imagining that day at the beach. If you're like most women, exercise isn't typically associated with enjoyment, feeling energetic, or having so much fun you don't notice time going by. Exercise, usually, is something you *have* to do; not something you *get* to do. It's another chore on your list, another hour (or two) out of your day. It's something that drains your energy and leaves you feeling not just tired, but exhausted.

I wish, as soon as you ripped open the cover of this book, I could've magically erased everything you've been taught about health and fitness and the messages that permeate the industry. In particular, I'd wipe out all the numbers you've been taught to use in valuing yourself, or simply for determining success.

As women, many of us have been conditioned throughout our lives to value ourselves on the basis of a number: a number on the scale, a number on the tag of our pants, body fat percentage, how many calories we ate today, how many calories we burned in our workout.

Many of us do this without even realizing it, especially if we're around other women who do the same thing. We'll sit and chat about what we hate about our bodies without once considering, "Could these things I'm saying be hurting me, or at the very least, be holding me back?" or even, "Why am I doing this?"

For many women, constant dieting, pointing out flaws, scolding themselves for eating too much, and gauging their worth by how good or bad they were at the dinner table or in the gym is just "part of being a woman." As for the negative conversations that obsess over body image and weight loss and how you need to diet harder, you may think it's just something women talk about—no big deal.

But in fact, those conversations feed a negative self-image and fuel dissatisfaction with your body. We think it's commonplace, and we never stop and ask ourselves whether it could actually be doing us harm. If you stop and reflect, you can see that talking this way does affect the way you think about yourself. The statements you make to yourself can be a tool either for putting yourself down or for building yourself up.

The way you talk about your exercise and eating habits and body can be self-defeating, or it can be self-empowering. It's all in how you *choose* to talk about it.

## LIFT LIKE A GIRL IN REAL LIFE

"The weight room really helped me let go of my body image issues. For me it was a mindset shift to striving to be more, instead of wanting to be less! It meant forgetting about losing weight, shrinking, eating less, and shifting to being unapologetically strong, adding muscle, and taking up space. In the past, all of my gym time and food I ate was calculated and measured, always with the goal of consuming less and making myself smaller. Once I started weight training, food became about helping my body recover and get stronger, and the gym became about being bold, instead of literally running scared on the treadmill. It doesn't matter to me if my stomach and hips feel bigger one day over the previous, because

I can still lift the same number of pounds either way and am making progress. This new mindset has helped me become more confident at work, and I've gotten a few promotions and raises since I started focusing on weight training a couple of years ago."

That's why the *Lift Like a Girl* methodology starts with strengthening your mindset, before you begin working on your body. The strength training programs and nutrition guidelines in later chapters will do amazing things for your body, but this chapter imprints the right tone and focus in your mind.

I know it can be difficult to change what you've heard and been taught to value over years, or even decades. Perhaps you're doubting the effectiveness of changing your mindset or think it's a ridiculous waste of time. But as you get away from the information targeted toward women—what's valuable, what's ideal, what's "fixable"—you'll be able to transform your mindset with ideas that are empowering and self-talk that is intrinsically motivating.

This chapter will rebuild your mental foundation. The way you evaluate your body against what's considered to be "ideal," the arbitrary numbers you use to determine success, the habit of viewing your body negatively, the belief that fitness has to be extremely complicated or time-consuming to be effective—this mindset and these thoughts have become unconscious habits.

To transform your mindset into a powerful tool that helps you achieve your goals, you must first create new thoughts. It starts with putting effort into being consciously aware of the thoughts and conversations we have about our bodies, and then changing and reinforcing them with productive thoughts and actions. With consistent practice, this empowered perspective will become your default lens; it will change not only how you view your body, but also how you view yourself.

## ANOTHER WOMAN'S BODY IS NOT YOUR MEASURING STICK

"I want to look like Jennifer Aniston," she said, pointing at the magazine cover. Those statements are what a personal trainer's nightmares are made of. When a potential client says she wants you to help her to look like another woman, it only means trouble.

In this example, I pointed out to the potential client that even Jennifer Aniston doesn't really look like the Jennifer Aniston on the magazine cover. She has a professional hair stylist, makeup artist, people that pick out the clothes that flatter her best, and photographers who use perfect lighting. Not to mention they still use photo editing to create the perfect, flawless image.

If we compare ourselves to professional, digitally altered photos of celebrities armed with a team of expert hairstylists, makeup artists, custom-designed clothes, and photographers, we're all screwed. We stand no chance.

At the same time, though, I understood where she was coming from. I've been there too. When I hated my body, I compared myself to other fitness women: "I love her arms. I love her stomach. When my body looks like that, then I'll be happy." When I realized what I was saying and the comparisons I was making, it stunned me. I was comparing myself to women who had a drastically different body type than me, women who had longer torsos and shorter arms and legs. There's no way I could look like them, because I have the opposite body type: short torso and long limbs.

Saying, "I don't like my body—I don't like what I have to work with. I want that; I want *her* body," was ridiculous. I can't make my body look like someone who has a radically different body shape any more than I can make myself look like a kangaroo.

It's like what happens when you want a new hairstyle. I've taken my stylist photos of haircuts I liked, only to have her tell me, "Nia, it's not going to work. You have fine hair, and hers is thick. Your face shape is longer; the one in the picture is more round. This haircut isn't going to have the effect you want it to. Your hair and face shape are different in every possible way."

Why do we keep comparing ourselves to other women? Why do we fight to achieve what society and the health and fitness industry have deemed "the standards"? Why have we passively absorbed these messages and allowed them to determine our self-worth?

In many ways, we do it without thinking about it. We've been exposed to these ideas through our moms' examples, or the magazines we read growing up, or the friends we've admired, or the comments we heard from peers in school. Like a sponge, we've soaked it all in; our brains have been saturated with this way of valuing ourselves, and we don't realize that many of our goals are externally based.

People do this every day without realizing that their actions are completely driven by the need, and desire, for approval from an external source. Like the woman who puts a post-workout selfie on social media, then checks every thirty seconds to see how many "likes" she received. While this woman may look, and be, incredibly fit, this mentality isn't healthy. Needing the constant approval from other people (and oftentimes total strangers) to validate your actions and serve as motivation isn't healthy. It's putting the power of how you view your body, value, and success into the hands of other people.

Someone saying you're beautiful doesn't make you more beautiful, just as their saying you're ugly doesn't make you ugly. Their opinion doesn't change who you are *unless you let it*. If they don't like something about you, that is *their* problem. It's not your responsibility to please them.

 Ambition means tying your well-being to what other people say or do. Self-indulgence means tying it to the things that happen to you. Sanity means tying it to your own actions.

—*Marcus Aurelius*

Fitness should not be about looking awesome to impress other people—whether it's social media connections, other people at the gym, or even your friends. Fitness means feeling awesome for yourself.

When we seek other peoples' approval, we don't realize what we're saying: "Their opinions about how I look matter more than how I feel or think about myself. It matters more than my being who I really am or determining for myself what matters."

Giving other people the power to build up your sense of worth is inviting them to tear it down later.

I've had ample experience with this. I'm not a "girly girl," but I did my best to play the part in high school because, according to my classmates, that's what girls were supposed to do. You're supposed to dress girly. You're supposed to wear makeup. You're supposed to act a certain way so the boys like you.

Even though it made me uncomfortable, I crammed myself into that mold. I did the hair, I wore the makeup, I put on the (occasional) dress, because what other people thought of me was supposed to be the most important thing. I needed people to like me, approve of me, tell me I did a good job. I allowed external standards (i.e., the opinions of others) to determine my worth and set the standards I should strive to achieve. I never even thought of asking, "Is this something *I* want to do? Does this feel good to *me*?"

 Whenever externals are more important to you than your own integrity, then be prepared to serve them the remainder of your life.

—*Epictetus*

We do the same thing with health and fitness. How many times have you scrolled through a social media feed and seen people posting pictures of a workout, followed by a flood of comments and praise? Or the comments telling one of your friends how awesome she looks in her gym mirror selfie? It's easy to see those things and think, "Well, I guess I should look like that, because that's how you're supposed to look. Look at all the praise you get when you look this way."

We can't control what anyone thinks about us—positive or negative, better or worse, like us or hate us. What we can control, however, is what *we think* and what *we do*. We can decide why we're doing what we're doing, and whether it's truly making us happy.

You can, and should, set your own standards and take the time to discover what matters most to you.

## WHEN THE NUMBERS DON'T ADD UP

While some women are trying to attain the specific images of what "fitness looks like," others are trying to get back to a previous version of themselves. The picture they have in mind isn't from a magazine—it's from their high school or college yearbook.

But even a picture from your past isn't a good measuring stick for success. That's because our bodies and priorities change with time. You might have been more physically active in college because you were on a sports team, but now working your dream job keeps you sitting behind a desk all day. Maybe when you first got married you had ample time to work out with friends, but now you have kids and a jam-packed schedule that makes it tough to get to the gym.

Rewinding the clock isn't an option for anyone. Fortunately, though, your health and success aren't defined by the previous version of you. They're defined by the actions you take today.

Here's an example you can likely relate to:

A woman hired me because she wanted to lose the excess weight she'd accumulated over the years. She was dead set on getting down to 140 pounds, because that's what she weighed in college, and it was the weight she thought would allow her to finally love her body. This goal weight is an example of an obsessive, absolute, outcome-based goal. She's basically saying, "I better reach 140 pounds—anything else makes me a failure."

Rather than chasing that number, I had her focus on *the actions* that would lead her in the direction she wanted to go (less fat and more muscle, so she could get the toned look she wanted). After a few months of consistent strength training (which you'll see how to do in chapter 4) and following simple nutrition guidelines (which you'll receive in chapter 3), she felt incredible. During our training sessions, she'd rave about how good it felt to be strong, how much confidence she had, how much she enjoyed getting stronger, how her clothes were looser and she had to buy new ones to fit her changing shape, and how she saw muscle definition she didn't know she could even have. Or, as she put it, "I feel like I'm discovering new muscles!"

Then one day she walked through the gym doors, and the energy and excitement she normally displayed had completely vanished. Something had happened.

That something was stepping on the bathroom scale that morning for the first time in months. She "only" lost five pounds. (When we started working together she weighed 160 pounds and was now 155.) "I don't get it," she moaned. "I feel great, my clothes fit better, I love my workouts, and I look different, but I'm still so far from my goal of 140 pounds."

Do you see the glaring problem here? The huge disconnect between what the bathroom scale said and what actually happened?

The scale is not revealing what happened over the past several months! The scale only displays a five-pound loss, but she's radically changed her body composition. She lost more than five pounds of fat, but she also built muscle. The scale doesn't tell you that. The scale doesn't say, "Hey, you weigh five pounds less, but you actually lost fifteen pounds of fat and added ten pounds of fat-free mass. You've improved your body composition, and even though you've 'only' lost five pounds, you look different because muscle is more dense than fat—that's why your clothes fit looser. To tell you the truth, I have no idea why you're allowing me to affect your mood or determine your success, because I just show you a number—*you* are in charge of interpreting what that means."

This is why you shouldn't rely on the scale to determine your success. As I reiterated, the number she's chasing shouldn't matter, because, according to what she said, she looks awesome, feels fantastic, and for the first time is enjoying her health and fitness lifestyle.

There's a place for the scale, especially for someone who is very overweight. The important thing is to look at the scale *objectively* and to remove all emotion from the number you see.

If you're going to use the scale, remember the following:

- Use the numbers as raw, objective data. The number you see should have no influence on your sense of self-worth.
- Know that the more weight someone has to lose, the faster they can lose it. The less weight someone wants/ needs to lose, the slower the rate of fat loss should be (to prevent/limit loss of muscle).
- If you choose to track your bodyweight because you want to lose weight, weigh daily at the same time, and take a weekly average. The weekly average is what you should track, because it's more accurate since daily weight can fluctuate for any number of reasons.

In addition to the scale, there are other important markers worth tracking: blood pressure, blood panels, how your clothes fit, improving your performance in the gym, energy levels, consistently applying the simple nutrition guidelines, and so on. If you're the type of person whose mood for the entire day can be affected by the number on the scale, stay off of it and track these things instead.

---

This story is a prime example of how self-defeating an absolute outcome-based goal, like an "ideal" weight, can be. A number is just a number—it's only one potential marker of success, and not always a very good one. It doesn't tell you everything else that's going on. You're better off focusing on the actions that lead to results and how you feel—things that matter more than an ideal number you've been convinced is important.

The problem with the woman just mentioned and others who chase a specific number (e.g., a goal weight or even pant size) is the disconnect between the changes they feel and see, and the standard they've got in their head. The problem is a focus on an arbitrary number—allowing the number staring at them from the scale to elicit an emotional response and determine their mood for the day.

 Your best weight is whatever weight you reach when you're living the healthiest life you actually enjoy, and if more people embraced that definition, I'd wager we'd see more success than we do watching people serially suffer.

—Dr. Yoni Freedhoff

It doesn't have to be that way.

Now, prepare yourself, because I'm going to share a shocking fact with you: Every one of us is going to die.

That's not a welcoming thought, but it's a fact nonetheless. We all have the same ending. Once that ending arrives, I know I'd rather not look back on my life and see the years spent struggling to attain some ideal bodyweight or clothing size that added no value to my life. I'd rather, instead, be proud of building a strong, healthy, functional body that served me and allowed me to live my life to the greatest possible extent.

Wouldn't you?

A health and fitness lifestyle should make you and your life better—it shouldn't be something you revolve your life around.

## QUIT THE COMPARISON GAME

With the debut of every summer Olympics, I can always count on the appearance of fitness articles with headlines like, "How to get abs like the US gymnastics team!" You've seen them, no doubt. Heck, maybe you read them for the irresistible "secret tips" they promised to reveal.

Let's take a step back and ask ourselves how much sense it makes to compare our bodies to sixteen- to twenty-year-old professional athletes who spend at least thirty hours per week training for their sport. Exercise, essentially, is their full-time job. They're not only talented, the cream of the crop, but they're genetically inclined to excel at these sports, due to their body type.

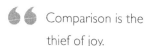

> Comparison is the thief of joy.
> —*Theodore Roosevelt*

And let's not forget that the physical appearance of these gymnasts is a by-product of their training. They don't train for thirty hours each week because they want a defined midsection or sculpted shoulders—they look that way because of their training and nutrition regimen. Their physical function has led to their physical form.

Don't compare yourself to anyone, especially to professional athletes who not only train exceptionally hard, but likely have a genetic advantage. Admire them, yes, for discovering what their bodies are capable of doing, for working hard to excel at their sport, and for their grit, dedication, and perseverance. But no one else's body should be your measuring stick for success. There is no "one size fits all," because everyone's genetic makeup is unique. Every body is different, and yours is no exception.

If your body isn't conforming to the shape or size you want it to be (or you've been told to strive for), at some point you have to stop blaming yourself. You didn't get to choose your genetics—whether it's wide hips or no hips, big boobs or small boobs, short or tall, thin or predisposed to obesity, it's what you have to work with.

Instead of pursuing a futile, absolute, external standard (e.g., I want abs exactly like hers), let's take a sober look at reality. I had to do the same thing, and that meant saying, "I'm going to start over and focus exclusively on getting stronger. This is my body, so I'm going to see what it can do. I'm going to discover the unique strengths it has."

There are two potential sides to health and fitness. On one side, you have the common approach—it's all about dieting, eating less, losing fat, trying to shrink, exercising for punishment. This side is filled with minimizing words like *less, smaller, shrink* because we've been led to believe that they lead to satisfaction and happiness. This is the side most women are familiar with.

On the other side, we have something vastly different. On this side, we forget about fat loss (or at least stop making it the most important goal), and focus on getting strong with a few basic exercises. We refuse to use exercise as punishment, and instead let each workout be its own reward. We forget about decreasing the weight on the scale, and instead set our sights on increasing the weight on the barbell. We forget about avoiding foods, and instead focus on all the things we can eat that make us feel awesome. On this side, we embrace words like *grow, strong, empowered, confident, more.* This is the *Lift Like a Girl* side and, as you'll soon discover, it's absolutely awesome.

Think for a second about whether focusing on less has really worked for you. Has it made you happier? Has it helped you like your body more?

If not, then how about this...

Screw *less,* and choose to become *more.* It's fun, it's empowering, and it's likely an approach to health and fitness you've never considered. Once you commit to it, you're going to love how becoming more means more of who you really are. More of the rewards that mean something to you. More ability to live your life the way you want to. More confidence to build the future you want.

I know it's a radically different mindset to focus on getting strong and eating more of the things that make you feel great instead of chasing a smaller number on the scale and trying to avoid certain foods you've been told are bad—to stop comparing yourself to others (or a younger version of yourself) and instead to become the best version of you. It may be intimidating, but once you declare, "Screw *less,* I'm going to become *more,*" you'll be shocked to discover how good it feels to be not only strong, but free from the burden of trying to be less.

The way you eat and move your body shouldn't be about trying to look like someone else or sculpting a social media-worthy body or thinking you'll only be happy if you look a certain way. It should allow you to discover, and appreciate, the incredible things your body can do, and you should want to do even more.

# WHAT REALLY MATTERS TO YOU?

When was the last time (if ever) you stopped and asked yourself, "Why do I eat the way I do? Why do I work out? Why do I want to eat better and work out? If it's not to try to look how other people expect me to look, or to look the way I feel obligated to look, why do I do it?"

Changing your thoughts and actions starts with understanding your motivation and "whys." That's where your action-based goals should start. Then, as you're rethinking your mindset, put your energy into the actions that can make you feel good right now: performing three workouts a week; making simple, smart nutrition changes; changing the conversations you have about your body; improving how you respond to bad days and choices that don't benefit you.

> When you approach health and fitness the *Lift Like a Girl* way, you can start feeling great about yourself right now. It's about creating a sustainable lifestyle so you can enjoy the process, not just the results it provides.

Actions alone create results. So that's where your focus and effort should go.

Embrace the action-based mindset with health and fitness. Focus on getting stronger by performing three workouts per week, and you'll feel and experience the effects for yourself. Add more weight to the bar, have fun by improving your performance each workout, and don't be surprised when you actually enjoy your workouts, because you finish feeling energized, not defeated and exhausted. Make simple nutrition changes, and eat meals that leave you satisfied.

These are the actions that lead to the results you want.

Actions allow you to focus on the here and now—this moment. Why is this important? Because the present is what you can control, using lessons learned from the past that lead you to the future you want to create.

When you focus exclusively on performing these actions consistently, you will notice your clothes fitting better. You may even exclaim as so many have, "Oh my goodness, I saw a new muscle today! Things are happening!"

Those feelings, combined with your experiences with strength training in the gym, will go with you outside the gym too. With progressive strength training, women begin to feel more appreciative of what they can do with their body in their daily lives. They enjoy the small things like picking up their kid, hugging their partner, playing with their dog, and being able to perform other tasks of daily living with greater ease and confidence. They also take the strength and confidence built in the gym into their personal and professional lives, as well.

## LIFT LIKE A GIRL IN REAL LIFE

"I spent a few hours moving chunks of concrete by myself since the spouse had to work. It involved squatting and lifting heavy chunks of concrete from the ground up to the pickup bed. Once I got to the concrete recycling place, we had to throw them from the back of the pickup to the pile. I had no problem lifting any of it or tossing it to the pile. The guy working at the dumping place even commented on how fast I was."

Action-based goals—such as scheduling three workouts per week on your calendar, or making sure you have a good source of protein with all meals—give you a great place to start making the changes in your mindset. It's about performing these small actions and building upon them. You don't have to look at the scale and think about how far you have to go. Think about the actions that have a cumulative effect and lead you in the right direction.

If you're skeptical about this approach, just try it. Get into the process of exploring a different aspect of health and fitness from what you've tried before, and see what happens. So often we have self-imposed limitations on our value and abilities that we never realize were put there. But once you take that first step, you'll start discovering all the things you've never considered were possible.

## ARE YOUR GOALS RATIONAL OR OBSESSIVE?

Remember the woman I told you about earlier who loved the changes in her body, but was quickly deflated when she stepped on the scale? When so much value is placed on absolute, specific outcomes (e.g., "I have to reach my goal weight of X"), you overlook what you have accomplished, including the positive changes to your body. That's the danger of saying, "I want my pre-baby body back. I want to weigh what I weighed in high school." You're blinding yourself from seeing what you are doing well, what you achieve, the habits you're establishing, all because you're fixated on a specific outcome.

If I fought my way back to what I weighed in high school, I would have to drastically limit my daily calorie intake and work out much more frequently. And I'd feel horrible. Maybe I'd be able to say, "Yay, I reached my goal weight," but I would feel like a steamy pile of poo, and it would be a constant struggle to maintain that weight.

Reaching a goal weight is meaningless if the lifestyle demanded to achieve it is miserable, especially if you could look and feel amazing at a bodyweight that's simple to sustain long-term. We'll talk more about this in chapter 2.

I understand why we place so much value on a specific number on the scale, or have an indelible image in our minds of what a "good weight" should look like. We can't expect to have a history of comparing ourselves to other women, disliking our bodies and viewing exercise as punishment, or allowing our happiness to hinge upon reaching a specific bodyweight and then expect to erase that long history in a single day, or even a month.

Just as you must strength train consistently to get stronger and transform your body, so too you must strength train your mind regularly if you want noticeable, lasting results.

That means setting rational goals about being healthy and strong, rather than obsessive goals about your appearance. It's the difference between wanting to get stronger and feel incredible, and lusting over an elusive six-pack. If you have a lot of progress to make to improve your health or revamp your mindset, you have to understand that it demands consistent action. You must practice the actions that lead you where you want to go, and learn to stay motivated with the rewards they provide along the way.

Creating this new, powerful mindset takes perseverance. You can't just say, "Today I'm going to be grateful for something my body can do and focus on rational goals," and then tomorrow skip that step. Habits aren't formed by simply deciding; they're forged from consistent, frequent, deliberate practice.

Once I decided to focus on my body's strengths instead of obsessing over what I disliked, I didn't just wake up one day loving my body for what it could do. It was a pragmatic process of taking action in ways that allowed me to love my body a little more every day.

Here's how you can tell the difference between a rational goal and an obsessive goal:

- An obsessive goal may be based on external standards (e.g., sculpting the perfect butt because butts are an "it" body part to flaunt and will get you more attention).
- A rational goal is based on internal factors (e.g., doing something because it feels good, or because it makes you a better version of yourself, such as working toward deadlifting one and a half times your bodyweight).

- An obsessive goal demands a specific outcome. For example, "I'm going to reach my goal weight of X so I'll fit in my old jeans and people will think I'm hot."
- A rational goal says, "I'm going to improve my health and get stronger because I want to be able to move better and have a higher quality of life. The physical transformation will be a side effect, a bonus."

- An obsessive goal is all about the destination: achieving a final outcome.
- A rational goal puts the focus on the process itself—the actions you must take repeatedly. Setting a rational goal means saying something to the effect of, "I want to be leaner, and a flat stomach would be nice, but I'm going to focus on the actions that will make me stronger, improve my health, and make me feel fantastic, so I create a sustainable lifestyle to ensure I maintain the results I achieve."

## FOCUSING ON MORE

If you've been struggling against the body you have, it's paramount to accept where you're at, right now. You can't have different parents, longer legs, or a different genetic makeup. This is your body—whether you love it or hate it or simply don't know what to think of it.

Your journey may be significantly harder than others because of your genetic predisposition, but swapping out your reality isn't an option. What you can do—really, the only thing you can do—is make the most of the reality you have.

I'm not going to delude you and say, "Just love your body. You're unique and perfect just the way you are." That kind of *Poof! Feel better!* rhetoric is stupid, not to mention condescending. I know from experience that instantly loving your body and breaking free from bad habits doesn't work that way, at least not for most women.

Whether you dislike your body or want to love it even more, getting there requires action. It starts with accepting your current starting point. Most of us hone in on our weaknesses—pain or injuries that prevent us from doing certain exercises, struggling with movements that used to be easy, a "failure" to be consistent with nutrition changes—thinking that in order to improve, we must identify everywhere we slip up.

In reality, all this calling out of weaknesses makes us ignore our strengths. You may even have strengths you've never taken the time to discover.

As a personal example, when I realized I was comparing myself to women who had a completely different body shape than me, I said, "This is ridiculous. I'm just setting myself up for failure, and I feel terrible about myself. Screw that. I'm going to make the most of what I have to work with. I'm going to discover what my body is capable of doing, and becoming, in its own unique way."

When I shifted my focus from obsessing over the traits I didn't like about my body, fixating on my perceived weaknesses, and chasing obsessive, outcome-based goals to discovering what my body was capable of doing, I found out that I'm naturally good at deadlifting. It's an exercise my body is built for, thanks in part to my long arms (long arms are an advantage to deadlifting because the bar travels a shorter distance).

As my friend Dr. Krista Scott-Dickson says, "Strengthen your strengths." And that's what I did. I decided to make the most of something I was predisposed to excel at. Rather than fighting against my body, I worked with it and highlighted its natural abilities. The first time I pulled 225 pounds (that's two forty-five-pound plates on each side of the bar: a fun deadlifting milestone), I was elated. I went on to pull 250 pounds (which equaled a double-bodyweight deadlift) for several reps. At my best, I deadlifted 300 for a set of three reps, and my best single was 330 pounds. That was more than two and a half times my bodyweight.

Focusing on what your body can do, and then doing more, does wonders for your mind, and it makes working out fun. And, yes, it leads to a physical transformation too.

I often refer to my gym time as "barbell therapy." When you have one of those days in which it seems like anything that could go wrong does (your alarm doesn't go off, the dog threw up on the rug...and you stepped in it, the car doesn't start), or you feel overwhelmed, pour that energy into your workout. People ask me if I meditate to alleviate stress. I do. Quite frequently, in my garage, with a loaded barbell.

Strength training is an amazing outlet for alleviating stress and frustration. When I'm having a crazy day and my brain is going bonkers, I lift. That energy gets released, and I walk away feeling relaxed and productive. It's a rewarding feeling.

My clients echo the same experience. Especially the ones who are busy—business owners, women with big families or demanding jobs—report that their gym time has become their "me" time, a priceless time in their day when they can discover what their body can do and focus exclusively on themselves.

## CHANGES YOU CAN FEEL

When you first start strength training, you'll quickly notice that you begin to carry yourself differently. You feel muscles you never really knew were there. Your body feels different, in the best way imaginable. You sleep better. Your mood improves. You have more energy. Your posture improves.

As these benefits accrue, daily life gets easier (and better) in the most surprising ways.

### LIFT LIKE A GIRL IN REAL LIFE

"Why I lift—a pallet of batteries came into work today. Each of the twenty boxes weighs about thirty pounds. I had to move them onto a cart, then from the cart to the shelf. A few years ago this would have left me out of breath and sore in my back and shoulders. These days, I can safely toss them around however I like! No sore back, no achy shoulders, just pure badassery! My bent over rows are going to feel easy-peasy this afternoon!"

Women have told me that when they go to the store now and a salesperson asks, "Ma'am, do you want me to help you with that thirty-pound bag of dog food?" they answer, "No thanks, I got it," throw a bag over each shoulder, and walk out. Others with manual-labor jobs—in warehouses or on farms— tell me they're carrying five-gallon jugs of water, sixty-pound sacks of feed, or bales of hay like it's nothing at all.

Women who had nagging aches and pains find those symptoms decreasing, or even disappearing (this is one instance when *less* is desirable). Moms with kids discover they have more energy at the end of a long day to chase their kids around. You'll even set a new one-trip max. You know what I'm talking about: You get home from the grocery store and want to get everything inside in the fewest possible trips. You load bag after bag on each arm and, before you know it, you're toting ten bags at once. So what if you forgot to unlock the door first and your hand is shaking uncontrollably as you try to slide the key in the lock? You set a new one-trip max.

## LIFT LIKE A GIRL IN REAL LIFE

"My husband and I were discussing our workouts the other day, and I was sharing how excited I was that the weight on the barbell kept increasing, as well as the dumbbell weight. He looked at me and asked, 'Right, and you don't have any shoulder pain any more, do you?' I used to have terrible migraines and deal constantly with shoulder and back pain from auto accidents. Since I started your total body program, not only do I not have that pain, but I've essentially eliminated shoulder-related migraines. Not only can I lift more and do more, but I am pushing myself to accomplish more as I never have before. Those extra pushes have eliminated chronic pain and fatigue in a way I never imagined. In short—thanks. Your simplicity and common-sense approach are not only valuable on a level of muscular strength and ability, but as a treatment for chronic, life-altering ailments as well."

Some women think I exaggerate the power of strength training—its power to make them a stronger woman—until they actually do it. They're astounded to discover abilities they didn't know were within them. It's like they're learning their bodies in a new way.

That's what fitness should be about: building a healthier, functional, stronger body that serves you and makes your life better.

Perhaps you think, "Great, that sounds wonderful, but I *still* want to get leaner and look better." I assure you that the workouts and nutrition information in this book will make that happen. Getting stronger with some of the best exercises you could possibly perform and following simple nutrition guidelines you can sustain long-term will undoubtedly transform your body. Regardless of whether you want to lose body fat or need to build muscle, I urge you to focus on what your body can do instead of how it looks. You'll be amazed at how it changes your life.

## SIMPLE STEPS TO BE MORE

It's the same reaction every time I train a woman to perform her first, unassisted chin-up—once she releases her grip on the bar after completing it, her face is glowing. Until then she had never performed a chin-up; she thought it was a goal that was out of reach. But when that self-imposed limitation is annihilated through consistent training, the empowerment is written all over her face. She exclaims, "Holy crap, I did it! I didn't think I'd ever be able to do that. What else can I do?" Then she's ready for a new challenge.

If you're used to measuring success with the scale or how you compare to a past version of yourself, you know how well that works (or more likely doesn't work). Try a different way—the *Lift Like a Girl* way—and see what happens. Put away the pictures, erase the ideal numbers, and ditch the absolute standards and goals. Instead, trust the process and see it through. Find out for yourself what's possible when you stop basing your happiness on numbers—be it body fat percentage, weight, bra size, age—and instead focus on the actions that build you up, make you feel good, help you live a life you enjoy, and reduce your stress.

Choose, in every way possible, to be *more*.

The *Lift Like a Girl* mindset is all about awareness. Again, your thoughts and actions are the only things you can control. Is what you say to yourself helping your goal for better health and being the best version of yourself, or is it harming it? Are the goals themselves helping or hindering?

As an example of being aware of what you say to yourself, one of the first guidelines I give my clients is to drop the "good" and "bad" food terminology (we'll get into this in depth in the nutrition chapter). No food is bad, or evil, or dirty. There's just food.

It's important to catch the comments we make to ourselves,

and change the conversation if necessary. For example, a woman may eat a cupcake and immediately after say, "Oh my gosh, I ate a cupcake. I failed to follow my diet again. I can't believe I did that. I screwed up and ate something dirty."

No. That is not an appropriate response. The solution begins with catching those self-defeating conversations early, and changing them or cutting them off. Instead of, "I ate a cupcake; I failed again. I can't do anything right," she should say, "I ate a cupcake." End of story. Don't extrapolate. She can choose to let that event be over with and move on. She needn't berate herself for eating a damn cupcake. The cupcake can just be a cupcake—why turn it into anything more than that?

> Your internal dialogue can build you up, or tear you down. Actively be aware of what you say to yourself.

Commit to maintaining a conscious awareness of your internal dialogue throughout the day, and change the conversations to something helpful and productive.

From putting on a pair of pants and looking in the mirror and saying, "I really don't like how my butt looks," to seeing an Instagram photo of a fit pro and thinking, "I want her abs"— stop those conversations from either escalating or starting in the first place. Once you catch yourself, ask, "What good is this doing? I'm not going to play that game. All it does is make me feel like crap. She looks good, good for her. I'm going to be over here and do what makes me feel awesome and moves me in the direction I want to go."

It takes time to transform your body; it's the same with your mindset. But the more consistent practice you put into building new, empowering habits, the easier these habits become. The more you consciously practice focusing on what you can control, taking action based on what matters to you, building your strengths and making the most of the body you have, the more that will become your default way of life.

You'll get to the point where you don't have to consciously monitor your thoughts to forge a positive mindset—it will just be what you do. And once your mind perceives things differently, positive changes to your body will follow suit.

A simple, pragmatic way to start is to spend time each day reflecting on three questions:

1. **WHAT DID I DO TODAY THAT MADE ME FEEL GREAT?**
   Instead of giving yourself a pass-or-fail grade based on how you ate or exercised, focus on what you did well and how it made you feel. Look through your day for things that surprised you in a good way. It could be something like, "That workout today was tough, but I did it and felt good doing it." Identify your strengths, and see if you can strengthen them further.

2. **HOW DID I BECOME *MORE*, EVEN IN A SMALL WAY?**
   Look for ways you broke free from the *less* mindset and did something that made you feel more awesome, more powerful, more alive. Maybe you ditched your obsession with burning calories for a determination to beat your previous workout performance. Maybe you let go of the diet mentality and enjoyed the heck out of a protein-rich meal that satisfied you. Be proud of these wins, and replicate them tomorrow.

### 3. WHAT WOULD I LIKE TO DO A LITTLE BETTER TOMORROW?

This question is not, "What did I do wrong? How did I screw up?" Do an assessment of the day, and look for an objective way to improve. It could be with your mindset, nutrition, or workout. For example, "When I looked in the mirror, I commented on how I hated the cellulite on my legs. Tomorrow, I'm going to be more mindful of what I'm saying about my body, and I'll cut those conversations short." Or perhaps, even though you ate a tasty, satisfying dinner, you later snacked on cookies, even though you weren't hungry. You acknowledge that if cookies are in the house, you're going to eat them. So that you don't have to rely on willpower to not eat the cookies at night, you plan to remove tempting foods from the house. When you really want a delicious dessert, you'll order your favorite at a restaurant or get a single serving and bring it home. This way you're not needlessly tempting yourself, but you're not depriving yourself either.

That's how you continue to become a better version of yourself: highlight, and enhance, your strengths. Look for ways to do a little bit better. Be objective and pragmatic.

Forging this mindset and honing these new skills will require consistent effort. But ask yourself: Do you have anything to lose by trying? Give this process a few weeks. After all, aren't you reading this book because you've tried everything else, or because you want a simple, sustainable lifestyle? You're already looking for something more, something

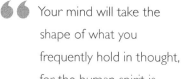 Your mind will take the shape of what you frequently hold in thought, for the human spirit is colored by such impressions.
—Marcus Aurelius

that works. Let me show you a path you haven't taken before.

I once heard someone say that you have to be aware of the information you take in, because what comes in is what forms you. That stuck with me. The thoughts we feed ourselves about who we are, what we're supposed to do, what we think about our bodies, who we want to become, and how we measure our value are important. And so are the conversations we have about our bodies with others.

> When people are complaining about their weight, pointing out flaws, or talking about how they need to diet harder, there are two ways you can respond:
>
> 1. Don't participate, or find someone else to talk to.
> 2. Better yet, do something unexpected: redirect the conversation. Blurt out, "Hey, want to know what I love about my body?" Maybe you love your strong legs, or perhaps (because you're following the Phase 1 *Lift Like a Girl* Program) you're now doing traditional push-ups and are ecstatic at the prospect of getting even stronger.

We can't change the entire culture we live in (at least not quickly), but we can immediately change the conversations we have with ourselves, and with others. You'll be building up not only yourself, but the other women around you too. You never know who these conversations can inspire.

---

What you read/consume with health and fitness will become your thoughts. This book will nourish you with good content. No bullshit. No ego stroking. No tricks or hacks. Just information that works and the encouragement you need to go a little farther, be a little more.

The key is not perfection, but perseverance. By feeding your mind useful information, you'll have the motivation you need to take action—the actions that make you more.

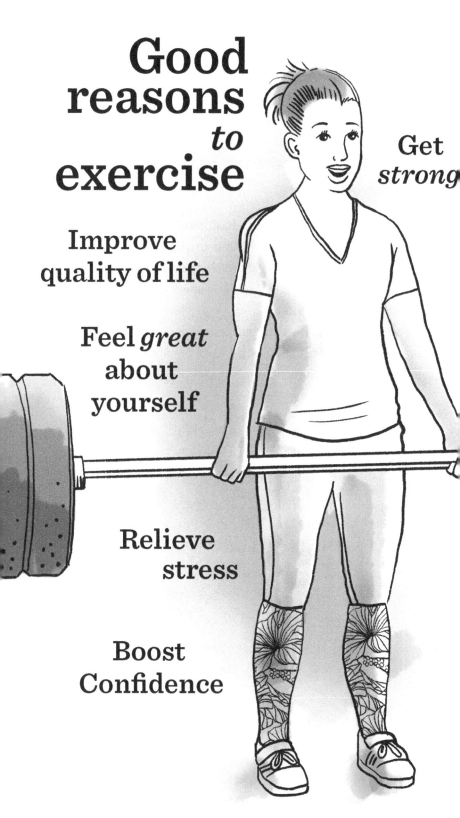

# CHAPTER 2

# Exercise Isn't Punishment

How many jumping jacks would you have to perform to burn off the calories from three chocolate chip cookies?

Answer: It doesn't matter. Because that's a stupid question.

Every holiday, the same recycled message appears. You see it on posters at your gym. You see it in social media memes. A photo of a delicious holiday treat—Thanksgiving pumpkin pie, Christmas cookies, Halloween and Easter candy—with a caption that shows the treat's calorie count, along with the number of miles you'd need to run or burpees you'd need to complete in order to burn off those calories.

Those messages exacerbate the mentality that we have to earn the food we eat. It turns every meal and snack into an equation. Women see something like their favorite cookies or Halloween candy and think, "Oh my gosh—how much exercise am I going to have to do if I eat one? Or two? Or three?"

You do not have to earn your food. You don't need a plan for burning off everything you eat. You don't have to calculate how long you'll need to strength train to burn off the mini-size candy bar you ate earlier in the day. You don't need to ask for permission to eat anything, nor must you justify your reasons for eating something.

All this "burn off what you eat" mentality does is mess with your mindset, as discussed in chapter 1. If you view your favorite treats that way over a long period of time, you start looking at all food that way: all or nothing, black or white, clean or dirty. "If you ate it, you have to negate it," your mind will start chanting. As shared in the previous chapter, that has the potential to lead you down a terrible path to disordered eating.

> Context and mindset are critical.

> It's one thing to choose to do a workout after a night of eating and drinking to excess because you know it's good for you to be active, and you're aware of the overconsumption. In this situation, you're making an objective, emotion-free decision.

> It's another thing entirely to view a workout as a deserved punishment because you think you're a failure and screwed up from overeating. This is an example of a subjective, emotion-fueled response.

> Similarly, performing a workout because you plan on eating a piece of cake for your birthday and you know a workout makes you stronger and healthier is different from thinking you can't eat cake unless you work out and earn the right to do so.

The former response is objective and rational, while the latter is subjective and driven by obsession, bad body image, and an unhealthy mindset. My experience with the emotionally fueled, body-hating, exercise-is-punishment mentality is what has led me to say, "Exercise isn't punishment, and you don't have to earn your food."

Context is important. Know why you're doing what you're doing, and change your mindset if needed.

## HOW WE MEASURE SUCCESS

Most women diet and exercise to reach a certain physical measure of success. After growing up and living in a barrage of marketing that tells women they're expected to look a certain way, women internalize the message and see exercise as a way to get there. Exercise isn't about getting healthier or stronger, or enjoying what your body can do, or building a body that makes your life better. It's about aesthetics, fixing so-called flaws, shrinking your body parts so you can fit into the next size down, or amplifying the "right" body parts.

By this measure of success, the one and only thing that matters is how you look.

As discussed in chapter 1, many women assume that reaching an aesthetic-focused measure of success means they'll be happier. But as I've seen too many times to count, even when a woman reaches her desired weight or clothing size, she's still not happy with her body and immediately looks for the next body part to improve, hoping that, perhaps, that goal will make her happy. "Well, my butt could be a little perkier. I really want washboard abs." She may have achieved the initial goal, but because she never stopped and appreciated what she already achieved, she quickly finds something new to obsess over.

Absolute outcomes (e.g., reaching that ideal bodyweight) are like a bottomless pit. Women keep throwing in their time, their energy, and their aspirations and wondering why the pit is not filling up. When they're not as elated as they expected to be despite losing ten pounds, they look for the next goal to chase or next flaw to fix.

The outside success doesn't translate to the increased confidence and happiness they expected. They're not looking at exercise as a way to feel good today or finding a fitness process they actually enjoy. They're doing it because they feel like they have to and don't know any other way.

As a result, diet and fitness end up being an endless cycle of stress, frustration, and guilt for many women. The infinite marketing messages that wearing a certain size or looking like a certain woman or fixing a certain flaw will bring happiness are hard to ignore. As a result, we go all in with the latest diet/ workout program, confident that if we do everything right, we'll get the outcome that makes us happy. But when something causes us to get off track—missing one workout or eating one meal that wasn't part of the diet—we try to make up for it the next day by working out extra hard and doubling down on food restriction. The makeup effort leaves us so exhausted that we're twice as likely to "cheat" again. After all, when a food is labeled "forbidden," we want it more than ever. It's just how our brains work.

A woman tries a new diet believing it will take her to the weight she wants. The diet says she can't eat this, that, or the other thing. She follows it religiously for a week or two, but then somebody brings cupcakes to the office or cookies to a PTA meeting, and she eats one. Immediately she regrets it and is stricken with guilt. The diet said don't eat cupcakes, but she did. What does it matter if she eats another one? Or if she eats the whole package? She's already screwed up; she might as well eat as many as she wants and get back on track tomorrow. Unless tomorrow is Saturday, in which case she'll continue to eat whatever she wants over the weekend, because who gets back on track on a Saturday? She'll start over on Monday.

She may get back on track, but she will inevitably "slip up" again and will be overwhelmed with guilt once more. She can't get, and stay, on track; she has to punish herself with an extra workout, and hopefully she won't transgress again. After ping-ponging back and forth for weeks, she finally gives up on the program. She couldn't stick to it as written—she failed to go all in—so she might as well quit. That is, until time passes and she tries the other diet or program that promises to be the solution.

That's the problem with these all-or-nothing, no-flexibility regimens. You either do everything correctly every time, all the time, or you screw up and say, "To hell with it." These programs promise happiness, but they're a setup for failure.

Change begins when you realize you can choose to get out of that cycle. You have the option of refusing to focus on the typical outcome-obsessed, all-or-nothing, one-size-fits-all rhetoric around fitness. You have the freedom to abolish that mentality and try a different, flexible, empowering method.

But it's a choice you have to make.

Scratch that—it's a choice you *get* to make.

## FROM TORTURE TO REWARD

When I was captive to the cycle of binge eating and plummeting self-image, working out was a tool of punishment: to burn as many calories as possible, to work out as hard as I could, as frequently as I could, and to atone for my binge eating sins.

Punishing yourself with grueling workouts or extreme restriction is not only unpleasant—it's not even helpful. When I accepted this truth, I was able to stop and ask how I could get back to where I used to be. Before the binge eating cycle began, I used to enjoy working out, and I loved strength training. I asked myself, "How can I make this fun again?" The first step was to stop going into every workout disliking my body and using exercise as punishment. Instead of looking at exercise as a tool to manipulate my body into some perfect ideal, I resolved to exclusively focus on getting stronger, and making it an enjoyable activity once again.

The fitness industry implies that happiness is a destination, one you reach at a certain weight or size or perfectly sculpted body part. But happiness is a *process*, one that builds upon itself every time you do something that makes you feel good in the here and now.

Not to get too philosophical, but let's think about it for a minute: Where does true happiness come from? Doesn't it come from doing your best to live up to your potential? From being the best woman you can be, and helping others do the same?

Happiness is a lifestyle—a process—not a final destination. And fitness is just one of the rewarding factors in the process.

Embracing this rewarding mindset involves stopping the punishment/restriction cycle and accepting the fact that the body we have is the only body we're ever going to get. Like it, love it, hate it, despise it, you're not going to get another one.

When you accept that, you can quit trying to torture yourself in order to fit an identity that other people say is right, or you've been led to believe will make you happy. You can stop trying to find happiness in an arbitrary number. You can let yourself commit to your own body, knowing it's the only one you have to work with, and resolve to make the most of it. When you approach fitness from that place of acceptance, that's when you discover that exercise can be enjoyable; it stops being punishment and starts being a reward. When you love how you feel, it makes you want to keep doing the things that make you feel good. No significant willpower required.

One of the best things I did that helped me love my body was to stop talking about wanting to love my body and instead put that energy into discovering what it could do. In the gym, that meant getting stronger. Then I didn't have to force it—it began to happen on its own because I looked beyond my physical form and focused on something deeper and, arguably, more meaningful and functional. The more I discovered how much my body was capable of, the more I genuinely loved my body.

Taking a new approach can be scary, even when you recognize that the familiar way isn't working (or it is completely dreadful). When I was battling disordered and binge eating habits, I was a trainer—I knew all these things in my mind—but I was terrified of breaking out of the punishment mentality that I'd lived by for several years. I was scared that focusing on getting stronger with just a few exercises wouldn't be enough. I was afraid that if I stopped punishing myself with extra workouts, I'd gain more and more weight. I couldn't extinguish that fear, but I did my best to silence it while I tried something new. I told myself, "You have to commit to this for a few months and see what happens. What's the absolute worst-case scenario in this situation? What you're doing now is not working."

That's one of the fascinating traits of our brains; we tend to inflate worst-case scenarios to extremes. But when we pause and take an objective look, we realize we've artificially pumped up these fears.

When I thought about my situation logically and rationally, I realized there wasn't a worst-case scenario. My fears were exaggerating the consequences of trying something new. Even though it seemed there was no way a less stressful approach could really work, I knew that my current restrictive approach only made everything worse. The only way forward was to simplify everything.

The only way forward was to simplify health and fitness. I had to transition from rigid rules to flexible guidelines. I started by stripping nutrition down to the bare minimum: the fewest guidelines needed to get me moving in the right direction. Same with working out: the fewest exercises that would give me the best results in my effort to get stronger. *Strength and simplicity* was my new mantra. Nothing else mattered. Instead, I would do the few things that must be done and not obsess over everything that could be done.

Prior to this new journey of simplicity and strength, I didn't realize how my focus on building a body I didn't hate was a self-defeating motivation. By saying, "I'll be happy when I look a certain way," I was admitting by default that I wasn't happy now. I had lost what I initially loved about fitness when I first began strength training as a teenager— the feeling of accomplishment, the pure joy that comes from building on my body's natural strengths, the satisfaction of improving my performance a little each time I repeated a workout.

I told myself, "I refuse to use exercise or strength training as punishment, in any context. I've got to look at training as an opportunity to get stronger, to discover what my body can do, and to see what else it can do as I go along."

Instead of doing numerous exercises that took an hour and a half to complete, I decided to focus on the fewest exercises that would give me the greatest benefit (you'll be introduced to these in chapter 4). Instead of concentrating on the size and shape of my body and trying to burn off the fat I loathed, the only thing I would concern myself with would be doing a little better every time I repeated a workout: doing one more rep than last time, or adding more weight.

## LIFT LIKE A GIRL IN REAL LIFE

"I absolutely love your no-nonsense, simple approach to fitness and nutrition, and I'm not exaggerating when I say it has changed my life. In the past I've also been obsessed with my eating habits and wanting to lose fat, and really overdid it with my workouts as well. I just couldn't understand how I could be working so hard and not seeing the results I wanted. Well, the last couple of years I've really been on the journey for the better. I've stopped obsessing about nutrition, and I've learned to stop trying to be perfect and just be happy with myself. I've been doing your training programs for the last year and a half and have seen more progress in that time than any other. In fact, just this morning, I finally hit ten straight chin-ups with neutral grip! That has been a goal of mine for a very long time. I have now come to love doing your minimalist programs and realized I don't have to end up in a puddle of sweat to make progress, or do twenty exercises."

At first it was difficult, and scary, to cut my workouts down so drastically. I was terrified at first: "I'm not doing enough. I'm not burning enough calories. I'm going to gain body fat." But when my brain would start to have those negative conversations, I would remind myself to change them. (Remember this from chapter 1?) I would remind myself that I'd been taking the "work out as hard as possible for as long as possible and limit your food intake" cycle for years, and it hadn't been working. "You have to commit to this," I'd tell myself. "Try it and see what happens—the most likely outcome is extremely positive."

After a couple of weeks of performing workouts that revolved around a few exercises with a focus on improving my performance, I noticed I wasn't as exhausted as I used to feel. I had, apparently, become accustomed to living in a constant state of fatigue—I was shocked by how good it felt to have energy left at the end of the day, and to finish a workout feeling accomplished and energized instead of depleted.

And by focusing only on my workout performance, I was starting to enjoy training again. Slowly but surely, I began to appreciate my body for what it can do and, at the same time, to develop a love for deadlifting, squatting, and pressing a progressively heavier barbell. I discovered that my body's anthropometry naturally made me good at deadlifting, and it excited me to strengthen that strength and see how far I could go with it. This "I'm good at deadlifting, so I'm going to become great at deadlifting" mindset was significantly more rewarding than trying to exhaust myself each time I entered the gym.

I started looking forward to my workouts, knowing I was going to be a little stronger each time. It allowed me to appreciate my body in an entirely new way, and the rewards kept accruing, even though I was doing less than I had previously.

Another bonus is that the positive benefits I enjoyed in the gym helped me outside of the gym too. I began developing a more positive mindset in other areas of my life. With that mindset, it slowly dawned on me that I didn't need to beat myself up, with workouts or anything else. I didn't need to punish myself when I wasn't perfect. I didn't have to be so hard on myself all the time.

Working out went from being a tool of punishment to being a tool of empowerment. It was something that built me up—physically and mentally—instead of tearing me down.

To be clear, this change didn't happen overnight. I didn't commit to changing, and then wake up the next day with a new outlook. I had to be intentional about each step in the process. For example, each time I went to the gym, I looked at my logbook for what I needed to do that day, and the only goal was to do a little bit better than last time. Once it was done, I was done. No more obsessing.

This positive focus in the gym carried over to how I approached nutrition. I still remember the first day I didn't binge after battling that habit for years. Where before I might have said, "So what? It's only one day," this time I told myself, "Yes! One whole day!" I made sure I celebrated each slow, steady step in the process.

This led to another revelation: how important it is to practice self-compassion. I've always held myself to a high standard in everything—I thought demanding perfection was a good thing. But now that I've experienced the dark side of it, I know demanding constant perfection isn't always helpful. I'm guessing, if you're like most women, you can relate. Like me, you've beat yourself up for falling short of an impossibly high standard. You've experienced how perfectionism can bring out the negativity in life, even in activities you used to enjoy.

Now and then, I encounter coaches who haven't gone

through this kind of struggle. When they work with women who are binge eating, they dismiss it with a quick-fix solution: "You just need to have a 'cheat' day during the week and stop thinking about it so much." This dismissive attitude makes women feel like they're broken—a lot of women won't even talk about their disordered habits and obsessive attitudes with their coaches because they're ashamed.

I've experienced the desperation, the fear, the sinking feeling that you're doing everything wrong. Please know it's not your fault that you feel this way. There are some things you've been told to do that led you down that path. It's okay to put your foot down and acknowledge that path doesn't work for you.

Many workout programs are like complete lifestyle shifts. They demand that you adopt a new wardrobe, a new way of speaking, and a complete identity makeover. That's the last thing I want to do with *Lift Like a Girl*. It isn't about replacing your identity; it's about enabling you to have the identity you want, starting with your physical fitness and health.

## MAKING IT MORE ABOUT YOU

When I talk with women about their fitness goals, once we get past the absolute outcomes, I hear the same comments over and over: They want to know their body serves them and lets them do the activities they want to do. They want less stress. They want to feel comfortable in their clothes. They want to have energy and time to do the things they enjoy.

They want health and fitness to be simpler. They want a lifestyle that allows them to develop a strong, healthy body that they can maintain without having to deprive themselves, obsess over food, or kill themselves in the gym.

That's what I created *Lift Like a Girl* to do for you. It starts with you evaluating what's important to you.

Some women say they've given up on fitness because they're burned out with how much time it demands. Most of the programs they've tried require spending hours at the gym, multiple days per week, and it's not practical for their schedule. It prevents them from doing other activities they love, spending time with their families, or excelling in their jobs. It makes them choose between feeling guilty for missing out on their lives and feeling guilty for skipping a workout.

It's not too much to ask for a healthy lifestyle to be simpler, to not be exhausting. That's why the programs in this book are designed to be as simple as possible. But the success of that simplicity starts with you. You need to make sure the body you want to achieve is a body you can maintain with a lifestyle you'll enjoy, because that's what *Lift Like a Girl* is all about.

If you think getting super lean will make you happy, you'd better be prepared to endure the lifestyle that's required to get it, and maintain it. But if you're miserable all the time, what good are those six-pack abs? Do you want your life to revolve around the gym and kitchen? Or do you want your gym time to revolve around living a life you enjoy?

We don't always think this through before we start a fitness program. I've seen it countless times with women who work with me—when they trust me and let go of absolute outcomes around weight loss or size and the need to do a traditional diet, they find that they can build a body they really like. It may, or may not, look the way they thought would make them the happiest. For example, I've had clients say they wanted to get incredibly lean, but they feel wonderful and love how they look at a higher body fat, *because the process that led to those results was enjoyable and sustainable.* They realize getting ultra-lean isn't the only possible outcome they could feel happy about.

That appearance-based outcome just doesn't matter the way it used to, now that they feel awesome, confident, and strong. They like how their clothes fit. They love the abundance of energy they have. Best of all, they're enjoying the process and are amazed that it takes less time out of their lives than they expected.

I love watching a woman's strength and confidence unfold, as she abolishes the unhelpful ideas about exercise and discovers how rewarding it can be to pursue health and fitness on her own terms. Often, her comments will start with something like this: "I'm finally confident in my own skin! My reflection in the mirror no longer controls me."

And a few months later she might say, "I just went from a size small shirt to a medium, and it was freaking awesome. I'm so proud of how much muscle I've gained in my shoulders, and my boobs are perkier now, too!"

Know this: Depending on your starting point, going up in size, or even bodyweight, is not a bad thing, if you look at why it's happening. That increase means you're doing awesome stuff.

It's worth pointing out that women who are overweight will likely drop in clothing size as they embark on the strength training programs, while women who are not overweight may stay the same size or even go up a size. It depends on a unique combination of factors—your strength training experience, your consistency, your starting point, and your genetic composition.

No two women will respond the same to strength training because no two women have the exact same body. Focus on getting stronger and improving overall health, and see where that takes you.

Let your body transform in its own unique way, and enjoy the journey.

Some women, on the other hand, do get smaller as they progress in the program. The changes in each woman's body depend on her individual genetics, her starting point, and what individual health looks like for her.

At the end of the day, if you feel more comfortable in your body, if you're stronger and have more energy and are kicking ass in your life, that's what matters. Not the number on the clothing tags or on the scale. Numbers do not define you.

One of my clients shared a personal revelation with me that I love: "Clothes are made to fit my body. I'm not supposed to make my body fit them."

These revelations happen all the time when you are

strength training, and not just about clothes. Another great story came from a woman who had visited a community pool where there was a sort of obstacle course—a rope strung from one end of the pool to the other, and "lily pads" you could walk across while holding on to the rope. She told me, "I never would have tried that before—I wouldn't have thought I was strong enough to hang on—but I had the confidence for it now."

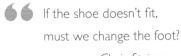 If the shoe doesn't fit, must we change the foot?
—*Gloria Steinem*

## LIFT LIKE A GIRL IN REAL LIFE

"Another win for working out. As I was leaving the gym this morning I heard a cry of alarm. I looked over and saw a woman on the ground between two parked cars. I went over and asked her if she was okay and if she needed help. She said she was good, but didn't look it. Again, I asked her if she wanted help getting up, and this time she said yes. She was just in such poor physical condition (or maybe she has a physical ailment) that she couldn't get up. I walked around the front of the car and took hold of her forearms and had her grab mine. I had to plant like I was deadlifting to get her up on her feet. It was a great lesson to me: Keep working out so you're not the one on the ground who can't get up!"

That's one of the greatest perks of strength training that people don't know, until they experience it for themselves. It gives you strength in areas that have nothing to do with lifting a loaded barbell. Lifting is fun, don't get me wrong. But a lot of women use it as a tool to be able to go out and do other things in their lives better. They try activities that used to scare them, and excel in situations that used to intimidate them. They're even able to stand up in moments when a tough choice is called for, and do the right thing for themselves. Their gains in the gym give them confidence to go out and live their lives, boldly.

Health and fitness—the *Lift Like a Girl* way—is supposed to make your life better. To help reinforce this obvious, but revolutionary, way of thinking, I've packed this book with stories that women have shared with me about how *Lift Like a Girl* has improved their lives in, and out of, the gym.

## LIFT LIKE A GIRL IN REAL LIFE

"My husband and I went for a cross-country ski. Last night, as I was putting on my gear, I discovered that I forgot my poles. Rather than not go, I decided to see how far I could get without them. I skied three of the five miles without poles, thanks to all those squats I've been doing. I'm pleased with how well I did uphill and down."

It's not up to a magazine or society or anybody else to tell us how we should look or how our bodies should perform. We get to decide. It's up to every individual woman to discover what health and fitness means to her. In doing so, she gets to discover that she's much stronger than she ever realized.

## DEFINING YOUR OWN SUCCESS

How do women begin to change what success looks like to them? It starts with pressing "reset" on the standards in your head. Instead of starting with what the media or the fitness industry have told you is the correct standard, embrace your own body as the standard. Whatever you've been taught to consider a flaw, or some part of your body you don't like, may provide a hidden advantage, if you'll only explore it.

 Define success on your own terms, achieve it by your own rules, and build a life you're proud to live by.

—*Anne Sweeney*

For example, I've worked with women who have what some call a "stocky" build: they're short in height, they have a proportionally long torso, and they have short arms and legs. "I hate my stocky build," one woman told me. But when they discover that their natural body structure makes them pretty damn good at hoisting weights, their thinking starts to change. They say, "Wow, I can keep adding weight to the bar. This is easier than I thought. I can get really good at this." What they once thought was a flaw is an advantage when it comes to certain exercises. Instead of chasing some ideal that is genetically impossible for them, they embrace the body they have and love it in ways they never previously explored.

Every woman's body is unique. Each should commit to discovering her personal strengths, and then build upon them.

The marketing around beauty and fitness has taught us to shrink (no pun intended) from words that invoke power and strength. As you get started on your personal *Lift Like a Girl* journey, it's important to distinguish what's true from what you've always been told. It's incredibly degrading that women have been discouraged from embracing words like "grow," "build," "muscle," and "increase." There's nothing wrong (or unfeminine) with an increase in your confidence, an increase in your energy, an increase in your physical strength and personal power.

Exercise, and strength training in particular, will no longer be punishment for missing a workout or making less-than-ideal food choices. It won't be something you do because you dislike parts of your body. And, I am hopeful, you will not look at it as something you have to do, but as something you want to do because of the myriad benefits it provides.

# Nutrition, *Simplified*

Eat mostly real foods

Get plenty of protein

Eat when hungry and stop when satisfied

Eat other favorite foods occasionally, *guilt-free*

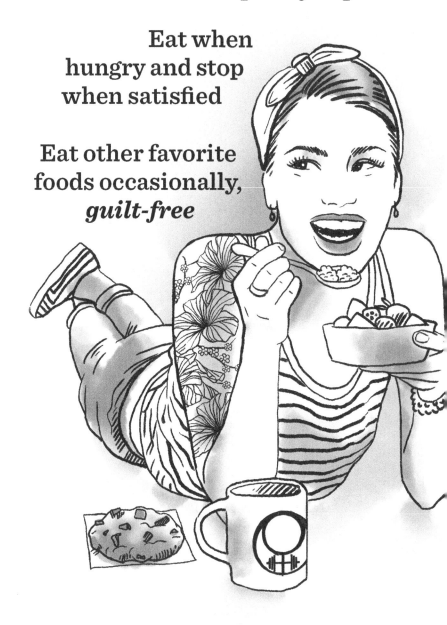

# CHAPTER 3

# Nutrition: It's Simpler than You Think

Several years ago, I had a consultation with a woman in her sixties. She shared her history and experiences with body image issues, relentless dieting, and bulimia. She started dieting when she was about twelve years old. As time passed and fashions changed around her, she tried countless diets, trying to get whatever that decade's "perfect body" looked like. But no diet ever worked the way she wanted it to. "I've never been happy with my body," she stated.

As the conversation progressed, my heart sank. This woman had spent decades without ever feeling content or comfortable in the body she had. She said her mom was a constant dieter, and she grew up assuming that being dissatisfied with her physical appearance and being on a diet was just part of what it meant to be a woman. She didn't know there was another way to live and eat.

It's tragic, but stories like this are not uncommon. My own stint with disordered eating lasted a few grueling years, but this woman—this incredible woman who had achieved wonderful things in her life—had been enduring her battle for several decades. The dos and don'ts that are shoved in our faces and blared in our ears no doubt contribute: "Here's how you can get pretty. Happiness is just a couple of pant sizes away, and this diet will get you there. Try this trick, avoid this food, fix this flaw, get smaller, then you'll be happy."

In high school, I had a big booty before having a big booty was "in" and deemed a worthy body part to flaunt. It speaks volumes to how fickle our culture is. A body part I was ridiculed for then was the same body part I was praised for later.

This is a prime example of why you should not allow others' opinions to decide how your body should look or what's "ideal"; it always changes.

The language and peddled gimmicks may have been different when this woman was younger, but the ideas stay the same—categorizing food as good or bad, diet- and figure-friendly or not, and evaluating ourselves based on how much of each category we eat or successfully avoid (and the ones we despise, but manage to choke down).

Nowadays, the popular food language is "clean" and "dirty." It may look like shorthand for how nutritious food is, but, as with exercise, the words we use about food matter in how we value ourselves and the actions we take. Such language exacerbates a distorted perception of food, and ourselves.

Think about it: If you eat a food labeled as "bad," what does that make you? It makes you bad. If you eat something "dirty," what does that mean? It means you screwed up because you ate something you shouldn't have.

Let's not forget the popular terms "cheat meal" and "cheat day" that accompany the dichotomous thinking. The idea behind "cheats" is that you follow your diet (whatever it may be) perfectly, and abstain from certain foods or entire food groups (whatever happens to be labeled "bad" or "off-limits" from the diet) most of the time. When the scheduled cheat meal or cheat day rolls around, you can eat all the "bad" stuff you avoided and couldn't eat otherwise.

It sounds innocent enough, and for some people, having a scheduled meal or two during the week when they can freely enjoy their favorite, not-so-healthy foods like pizza and ice cream helps them stay on track. They enjoy some of their favorite foods in moderate amounts, and then go back to eating minimally processed, nutritious foods without feeling deprived.

But for some people, it's not that simple. For some people, cheat meals create more problems than they were intended to solve. Here's an example I've heard innumerable times, and experienced personally: You go on a diet that has a list of "good" foods you can eat. A common example that became popular from the low-carb craze would be meat, poultry, fish, and non-starchy veggies (e.g., leafy greens, broccoli, cauliflower, asparagus), a little bit of fruit, eggs, nuts and seeds, and other low-carb foods. Anything else is off-limits, including foods like ice cream, baked goods, pasta and cereals, potatoes, pizza, and anything else that makes life worth living to people who love carb-rich foods. (People like me.)

Here's what is supposed to happen: You eat the allowed foods until the scheduled cheat day rolls around, then you eat whatever you want for that day. But here's what actually happens to many people: While you're being a good, low-carb eater, filling up on eggs, meat, veggies, and other low-carb foods, you can't stop thinking about your cheat day. Your work caters lunch unexpectedly, and it's from one of your favorite restaurants that has the best homemade cheesecake. Sadly, for you, you can't have a piece, because it's not your scheduled cheat day. You abstain, and pat yourself on the back for fully expressing your willpower.

Throughout the week your meals are pretty tasty and you enjoy them, but, my God, you would give your left pinky finger for a sandwich made with real bread, or a few scoops of your favorite ice cream. You even find yourself fantasizing about other cheat foods you don't really enjoy and typically would never eat. But now that they're forbidden, they sound amazing. Come cheat day, since that's the only time you're allowed to eat them, you're really going to eat them since you had to pass on your favorite cheesecake earlier in the week.

Finally, it's cheat day! You've been thinking all week about the foods you're going to eat today. You start off with baked goods for breakfast, and then an entire small pizza for lunch. You snack on things you don't even like, but you're eating them just because they're off-limits every other day of the week, so this is your only chance. By the time you're done with lunch, you're incredibly full, but you still have dinner and make sure it's something you can't eat any other day of the week.

The next morning, you don't feel too great. Typically, one of two things will happen at this point. One, in an effort to make up for overindulging yesterday, you eat as little as possible during the day. Two, you tell yourself you overdid it yesterday, so you might as well eat whatever you want today, too, and get a clean start tomorrow. The cheat day has now turned into a cheat weekend. Sometimes people get back on track the next day, but sometimes the cheat weekend even spills over into the next week, resulting in blowing the diet for an extended period of time. This is the all-or-nothing mindset in action: You're either following the diet perfectly, or you're not following it at all. I'm willing to bet I know the answer, but does any of this sound familiar?

This begs the questions: Why can people have drastically different experiences with cheat meals and cheat days? Why can scheduling a couple of cheat meals throughout the week help some people, while it can cause others to spiral into constantly thinking about food and going overboard when the cheat meal arrives?

It's comparable to the differences two people can have when standing on the bathroom scale. One person may see a five-pound weight gain and use that number as objective data and say, "Okay, it's time for me to get back to eating better and performing three strength training workouts per week." The other woman may see that five-pound gain subjectively and say, "Okay, so I've failed again. I'm never going to be able to reach my goals. I need to get stricter about what I eat. Time for two-a-day workouts."

Cheat meals are no different. For one person, it's an objective goal; they eat what they know is best for them during the week, and on the scheduled cheat day they moderately enjoy the other foods (or they schedule a couple of cheat meals spread throughout the week). But they don't force themselves to eat things they don't enjoy or try to limit.

For someone else, they spend copious amounts of time throughout the week planning their cheat day and constantly think about all the off-limit foods. Come cheat day, they don't just have two slices of pizza and a couple of scoops of their favorite ice cream. They eat *all the things* throughout the entire day, including stuff they may not even like. They justify these actions by saying, "I better eat all I can today, because it's back to my diet tomorrow, and I won't be able to eat these foods again until next cheat day." This individual doesn't enjoy foods in moderation—they eat a lot of it, well beyond satiety.

The second attitude is more common, in my experience. And it's why I'm not a fan of cheat meals or cheat days, because they can exacerbate bad mental and eating habits, and encourage overeating. They're also not as flexible. Sticking with the example above, if someone has a scheduled cheat day for Saturday, but their favorite dessert is offered to them on Wednesday, they can't enjoy it. And because they had to say no to something they truly enjoy, they end up eating way more foods that they don't even like later on.

And can we point out the obvious? The term *cheat* implies you're doing something wrong, forbidden, bad. And that's exactly the type of thinking we're trying to get rid of.

No two people are the same. What may help one person stay on track may amplify problems for someone else. Discover what works best for you. Don't force-feed (excuse the pun) a strategy if it doesn't work for you, or you don't enjoy it.

## DITCH DICHOTOMOUS THINKING

Several studies have examined the effects of black-and-white dichotomous thinking about food (i.e., labeling foods as good or bad, clean or dirty) and the rigid diet strategies they encourage. One study that examined the effects of flexible versus rigid dieting revealed a strong correlation with flexible dieting and an absence of overeating, lower body mass, and even lower levels of depression and anxiety. There was also a correlation that associated calorie counting and conscious dieting with overeating when alone and increased body mass.[1]

The research is clear and shows that rigid diets and dichotomous thinking about food isn't working for many people. Rigid dieting can increase the likelihood of eating problems,[2] while flexible control of eating behavior may be better for long-term weight control. And there's ample real-world experience to echo these findings.

---

1    C. F. Smith, D. A. *Williamson*, G. A. Bray, and D. H. Ryan, "Flexible vs. Rigid Dieting Strategies: Relationship with Adverse Behavioral Outcomes," Appetite (June 1999), *https://www.ncbi.nlm.nih.gov/pubmed/10336790.*

2    J. *Westenhoefer*, P. *Broeckmann*, A. K. *Münch*, and V. Pudel, "Cognitive Control of Eating Behaviour and the Disinhibition Effect," Appetite (August 1994), *https://www.ncbi.nlm.nih.gov/pubmed/7826055.*

Perhaps you've discovered this for yourself. Have you tried rigid diets, or attempted to only eat "good" or "clean" foods? How long were you able to maintain those eating habits before you gave up or became frustrated?

Studies also show that people who follow rigid diet strategies reported symptoms of an eating disorder, mood disturbances, and excessive concern with body size and shape. People who followed flexible diet strategies were not highly associated with BMI (body mass index), eating disorder symptoms, mood disturbances, or concerns with body size.[3] The study suggests that rigid diets, but not flexible diet strategies, are associated with eating disorder symptoms and higher BMI in non-obese women. Still another study revealed that black-and-white thinking around food (i.e., viewing food as good or bad, clean or dirty) may be linked to rigid dietary restraint, which impedes people's ability to maintain a healthy weight.[4] Dichotomous thinking could be a predictor of weight regain, as well.[5]

---

3   T. M. *Stewart*, D. A. *Williamson*, and M. A. *White*, "Rigid vs. Flexible Dieting: Association with Eating Disorder Symptoms in Nonobese Women," Appetite (February 2002), *https://www.ncbi.nlm.nih.gov/pubmed/11883916*.

4   A. *Palascha*, E. *van Kleef*, and H. C. *van Trijp*, "How Does Thinking in Black and White Terms Relate to Eating Behavior and Weight Regain?" Journal of Health Psychology (May 2015), *https://www.ncbi.nlm.nih.gov/pubmed/25903250*.

5   S. M. *Byrne*, Z. *Cooper*, and C. G. *Fairburn*, "Psychological Predictors of Weight Regain in Obesity," Behaviour Research and Therapy (November 2004), *https://www.ncbi.nlm.nih.gov/pubmed/15381442*.

A study in the *Journal of the International Society of Sports Nutrition* led by Alan Aragon, coauthor of *The Lean Muscle Diet*, examined the effects of different diets and body composition. Low-fat, low-carbohydrate, ketogenic, high-protein, and intermittent fasting can be similarly effective for improving body composition. No controlled diet comparison where protein and calorie intake is equal between groups has demonstrated a meaningful, fat-loss advantage.[6]

Why is this important? It means there is no "best" diet for fat loss. Any diet will produce weight loss if it puts an individual in a caloric deficit.

Next time you hear someone rave about losing weight on a new revolutionary diet, understand that happened because the diet put them in a caloric deficit. It's not magic; it's basic physics.

That's why one of the first steps in our new approach to nutrition is to ditch that language. It's time to quit assigning food into good/bad categories. Some foods should be eaten more often than others (more on this shortly), but it's time to

6    Alan A. Aragon, Brad J. Schoenfeld, Robert Wildman, Susan Kleiner, Tri-sha VanDusseldorp, Lem Taylor, Conrad P. Earnest, Paul J. Arciero, Colin Wilborn, Douglas S. Kalman, Jeffrey R. Stout, Darryn S. Willoughby, Bill Campbell, Shawn M. Arent, Laurent Bannock, Abbie E. Smith-Ryan, and Jose Antonio, "International Society of Sports Nutrition Position Stand: Diets and Body Composition," Journal of the International Society of Sports Nutrition (June 14, 2017), *https://jissn.biomedcentral.com/articles/10.1186/s12970-017-0174-y*.

change the terminology and eliminate the emotional baggage that frequently accompanies dieting tactics (e.g., "If I eat this, I'm bad").

The basis of the *Lift Like a Girl* nutrition philosophy is simplicity and sustainability. It's not just a means to build a better-looking body; it puts overall health at the forefront (cholesterol, triglycerides, etc.) and includes flexibility to suit your lifestyle and eating preferences.

Life should not revolve around what you do and don't eat. The ideal nutritional plan isn't a plan at all. Instead, it's a series of sustainable habits around eating that you don't have to think too hard about. You just do them because they make you feel great.

> A worthy goal with nutrition is to get to the point where you spend the least amount of time possible thinking about nutrition. You get there by first building simple, sustainable habits, and then practicing those habits consistently.

Thanks to our diet-obsessed culture and poor, or blatantly misleading, research touting "ultimate" diets, it takes a while to get that simplicity back (or experience it for the first time). To start, you must eradicate all black-and-white, good or bad, dichotomous language (and the thinking that goes with it) regarding what you put in your mouth. There's no clean, no dirty, no cheating. Nothing is forbidden or off-limits. Food is just food. Period.

If food is just food, then you are just you, no matter what

you eat. You're not a better person if you drink an organic kale smoothie or a worse person if you eat a tempura- battered, deep-fried candy bar.

However, one reason you're reading this book is because you want your body to feel better than it currently does, right? Whatever you're doing right now isn't working for you, and you want to make changes. You have to ask yourself what kind of changes have the best chance of sticking. The drastic, quick-fix kind? The rigid, all-or-nothing kind? My guess is that you've seen for yourself the ineffectiveness of those approaches. Let's scrap all that, and start over from a *more* mentality. Choose sustainable changes that are simple to follow, easy to adapt to, and give you more of the results you want every day.

Keep in mind that the goal with nutrition is to make changes today that you can continue practicing next week, next month, and next year. This is not a diet that concludes in twelve weeks—you're building a lifestyle. Don't overwhelm yourself by trying to change too much too fast. If you must, make one change at a time. This must become an enjoyable process—that's the only way you'll stick with it long-term, and that's the only way to achieve noticeable, lasting results with your health and body composition.

You only need three, simple, flexible guidelines.

## EAT MOSTLY REAL, MINIMALLY PROCESSED FOODS

Health matters most. Diets and eating plans come and go, but research has shown that the most important nutrition guideline that promotes health and helps prevent disease is to eat real, minimally processed, nutrient-dense foods most of the time.[7] They should be the foundation of your eating choices. Overall health matters, and eating mostly real, minimally processed foods (and thereby decreasing processed foods from your eating habits)—meaning predominantly plants—improves the nutritional quality of diet.[8]

As guidelines go, this one is rather boring and uncomplicated—it doesn't take much more than common sense to know what constitutes a minimally processed food. There's a huge variety: lean meat and poultry, fish and seafood, eggs, and dairy; and on the plant-based spectrum are nuts and seeds, beans and legumes, whole grains, rice, fruits and vegetables, herbs, spices, and healthy fats like olive oil.

The real, minimally processed guideline applies to all eating needs and preferences. Whether you're a vegetarian, vegan, pescatarian, equal-opportunity carnivore, or something in between, the same thing applies: eat mostly real, nutrient-dense foods.

---

7    James Hamblin, "Science Compared Every Diet, and the Winner Is Real Food," The Atlantic (March 24, 2014), *https://www.theatlantic.com/health/ archive/2014/03/science-compared-every-diet-and-the-winner-is-real-food/284595/*.

8    Euridice Martínez Steele, Barry M. Popkin, Boyd Swinburn, and Carlos A. Monteiro, "The Share of Ultra-Processed Foods and the Overall Nutritional Quality of Diets in the US: Evidence from a Nationally Representative Cross-Sectional Study," Population Health Metrics (February 14, 2017), *https://pophealthmetrics. biomedcentral.com/articles/10.1186/s12963-017-0119-3*.

Wondering what "real, minimally processed" actually means? It's food that takes the fewest steps possible to get from nature to your mouth. A potato is an obvious example. Another example is rolled oats—even though it's technically processed, it is still considered a minimally processed food. A lean, sirloin steak is minimally processed compared to a hot dog.

Minimally processed foods are usually single-ingredient foods, or a combination of them. For example, some store-bought spaghetti sauces include highly processed ingredients, but some include minimally processed ingredients like crushed tomatoes, peppers, onions, garlic, olive oil, salt, and spices.

There will always be some people who try to make this "real food" approach more complicated than it is. For instance, despite what you may have heard, there's no such thing as a negative-calorie food or a bad-for-you fruit or vegetable (unless you have an allergy). This is nonsense, and you should ignore it.

Despite what some so-called expert says, bananas will not make you fat. A caloric surplus is what causes weight gain. That can come from too many bananas, but it's more likely to come from too many high-calorie, nutrient-lacking, processed foods.

Rule of thumb: If a nutrition claim sounds bat-crap crazy (e.g., "Don't eat bananas because they make you fat," or "Sweet potatoes are superior to regular potatoes"), it probably is. Stick to the basics, and disregard the hyperbole.

Depending on what diets you've tried or the information you've been exposed to, some of the foods listed above may surprise you. Perhaps you've tried the low-carb approach, and so you're used to avoiding whole grains and potatoes. This is one problem with restrictive diets, especially diets that strictly limit, or eliminate completely, entire food groups. They're difficult to sustain long-term and can cause unnecessary stress, especially during holidays or with your social life.

Extreme restriction is not necessary, or helpful, for improving your health or body composition. No single food group or macronutrient is solely responsible for fat gain, nor are there any magic fat-burning foods either.

### LIFT LIKE A GIRL IN REAL LIFE

"I am SEEING the results in the mirror and in my measurements. My waist is down two inches! Two inches! In two and a half weeks. Thanks again for being a light in the often twisted and confusing darkness of the fitness industry. There's no need to ever read a "diet" plan or argue over calories, macros, or food restrictions. I eat food that makes me vibrant. I eat when I am hungry. I enjoy every bite. Seriously, I wish I could send your book to everyone who I know struggles with eating/dieting/weight loss/body images."

A simple, but powerful, nutrition mindset shift can be helpful as you follow this guideline. Instead of focusing on the foods you should eat less of (i.e., calorie-dense, nutrient-sparse, processed foods), focus on eating more of the foods you enjoy that are nutrient-dense, minimally processed, and make you feel great while contributing to your overall health.

Trying to give up foods you enjoy like fries, ice cream, pizza, and potato chips is likely to make you want them even more. Choose instead to focus on eating more nutrient-dense, minimally processed foods you enjoy. For example, include more vegetables and fruits in your meals and snacks. Whether it's adding diced veggies to your meatloaf, packing a few leaves of kale into a smoothie, adding a piece of fruit to your afternoon snack, or adding a side salad to your lunch, focusing on *more* instead of *less* will help this change stick.

A simple question to get you moving in the right direction is this: How can you eat more nutrient-dense, minimally processed foods you enjoy?

Side benefit: Not only does eating a variety of real, whole foods help you build a healthier body, but there's growing research showing promising results that eating real, nutrient-dense foods may help fight depression (partly by fighting inflammation and improving GI health).[9]

Resist any temptation to turn this flexible guideline into an unbreakable rule. The aim is to build sustainable habits that you won't have to think too hard about practicing. When you eat real, minimally processed, nutrient-dense food (e.g.,

---

9   Camille DePutter, "Mood Food: How to Fight Depression Naturally with Nutrition," Precision Nutrition (accessed October 27, 2017), *http://www.precisionnutrition. com/how-to-fight-depression-naturally-with-nutrition.*

good sources of protein, veggies, fruit, whole grains, etc.) most of the time, it makes it easier to enjoy your favorite processed or not-so-healthy foods on occasion, or when you really want them. When you're at your favorite restaurant that makes gelato so damn good you'd consider giving your left foot for a bowl of it, then eat it. If you love eating a ballpark hotdog at the game, get one. Enjoy these foods guilt-free. Then move on with your regularly scheduled habits.

It can be challenging to relearn the difference between diligently following a guideline and obsessing over it. It may be helpful to start with a soft target: the 85/15 ratio. Eighty-five percent of your food intake should be real, minimally processed, nutrient-dense food, and you can work your favorite foods that don't meet this guideline into the remaining 15 percent.

Now, some days may be closer to 80/20, and some even 95/5. That's fine. Don't obsess. If you discover a long streak where you don't get close to the 85 percent guideline, figure out what's going on, and get back on track.

How can you work in your favorite not-super-healthy foods (e.g., ice cream, pizza, etc.) into your eating habits? Let's look at a common example of someone who eats three meals per day. Over the course of a week, that's a total of twenty-one meals. The number of meals that would be part of the 10–20 percent where not-super-healthy foods can be worked in would be approximately two to four meals per week.

Remember, those two to four meals are not all-or-nothing opportunities. You're not eating forbidden or bad foods, so you don't need to gobble up as much as you can. And they don't have to be things like pizza or dessert or fried foods if you don't want them. You're simply being flexible and moderately enjoying some of your favorite foods. For example, instead of downing a small pizza all by yourself, halve the pizza and eat a side salad with it. This way you're still enjoying one of your favorite meals, but you're also making a nutrient-dense food choice to accompany it.

Have questions about carbs, and so on? Go to *www.niashanks.com/book-resource-guide/* for a free resource with great places to find science-based, nutrition information.

To sum up this guideline, think *more* with your food choices. More real, minimally processed foods that you enjoy. More true enjoyment of the occasions when you indulge in less nutrient-dense foods that you love.

## MAKE PROTEIN A PRIORITY

In addition to eating mostly minimally processed foods, make protein a priority with your meals and snacks.

Good sources of protein include lean meats, fish, low-fat dairy (e.g., Greek yogurt, cottage cheese, milk), eggs, and poultry—aim to include one of these minimally processed sources in your meals and snacks.

Many high-protein foods are from animal-based sources. If you're vegan or vegetarian (or simply want to eat more plant-based foods), include minimally processed, high-protein sources such as quinoa, lentils, beans, amaranth, tofu, and chickpeas in your meals and snacks.

The importance of protein, beyond one of its main roles of acting as a structural component of cells and tissues in the body, is that it helps you recover from strength training workouts (which you'll get in the next chapter). And out of all the macronutrients (fats, carbohydrates, and protein), it has the highest effect on satiety.

It's not uncommon for women to say they constantly feel hungry when dieting. The reason is often because they're not getting enough protein. To improve satiety and recover from your workouts, be sure to include a good source of lean protein in your meals and snacks. Or, to make this simpler, choose a protein source to build the rest of your meal/snack around.

Lean protein sources include skinless poultry, low-fat and nonfat dairy, fish and shellfish, protein powder, eggs, lean cuts of beef and pork (flank steak, sirloin, top loin, lean ground beef, tenderloin). Plant-based sources include lentils, beans, tofu, and quinoa.

Some fad diets in recent years have made protein the be-all and end-all. To be clear, I'm not suggesting you eat beef and plain chicken breasts at every meal. Remember, high-quality protein includes poultry, fish, eggs, lean meats, low-fat dairy, lentils and beans, or even protein powder if convenience is a priority in that moment. Start with protein as a foundation, and build the rest of your meal around it.

The combination of the first two nutrition guidelines—eat mostly real, minimally processed foods, and include a good source of protein in meals and snacks—combined with a progressive strength training program produces incredible changes in how your body looks, feels, and performs. You'll experience this for yourself soon enough. But there's one more helpful guideline.

Is this too much protein? No. It's safe to eat protein at every meal. The exception is if you have kidney issues, or you've been instructed otherwise by your doctor.

## EAT WHEN HUNGRY, STOP WHEN SATISFIED, BUT NOT STUFFED

The "eat when you're hungry and stop eating once you're satisfied, but not stuffed" guideline sounds simple enough. But it may take practice to get used to, or learn for the first time, depending on your starting point. I lost the innate ability to detect physical hunger from years of binge eating. Learning (or relearning, rather) to listen to my body again, to detect physical hunger, was a challenge. And I no longer knew what "satisfied, but not stuffed" felt like anymore.

What did help was slowing down, intentionally enjoying each bite. To be blunt, when I don't focus on eating slowly, I tend to scarf down my food, like a ravenous Rottweiler who missed a couple of meals. Eating fast tends to mean eating more—you're putting down one bite after the other until suddenly, you're not just full—you're too full.

Deliberately slow down, and enjoy your food more. The

more you practice this guideline, the easier it will become, and the less you'll have to focus on doing it. It will become a habit.

In addition to slowing down your eating pace, limit distractions while you eat. If you're eating in front of the TV or while working on the computer, it's more difficult to focus on the deliciousness in front of you. You'll finish your meal and realize you didn't taste anything.

If you're the type of individual who tends to eat beyond satisfaction, err on the side of eating less than you're used to, at least at first, as you relearn your body's satiety signals. Put less food in your bowl or on your plate than you usually would, and give your body time to process what it's been fed. Remember, you can always eat more later if you're hungry.

I'm not suggesting you develop neurotic practices like chewing a certain number of times before swallowing, or setting a timer between bites of food. Resolve to take your time when eating. It's okay to pause and give yourself a minute before continuing. It's even okay to leave some food on your plate. The feeling you're looking for is having your hunger satisfied while knowing you could comfortably get up and go for a walk.

American restaurants are notorious for serving humongous portions. If the entrée you order is more than enough, try to split it with someone. If that's not an option, commit to taking half of it home. This way you can enjoy socializing and having a good meal without overeating. Plus, you'll have a meal you don't have to cook or clean up after to eat later.

If the opposite happens—you eat too quickly, you put too much on your plate, you finish feeling uncomfortably full—don't beat yourself up. Learn from the experience. Take an objective look and ask, "Why did this happen?" Maybe you skipped breakfast so you loaded up your lunch plate because you were ravenous. Maybe you ate quickly while watching TV. Learn what you can from the situation so you can adjust next time.

To reiterate this guideline, strive to eat when you're hungry (when you're physically hungry and not bored, turning to food out of emotion), be mindful when you're eating, take your time, and stop eating when you're comfortably satisfied, but not stuffed.

This may take practice, but it's worth it.

## LIFT LIKE A GIRL IN REAL LIFE

"My mom just came back from a checkup and told me she's lost twenty-five pounds in the last five months, and over twelve inches from her waist. She's gone from a size twenty to twenty-two-plus to a twelve! Special thanks to Nia Shanks for providing such incredible information for me to share with her. I've watched her try and fail every year for the last twenty years. Thank you for changing our lives! My mom has tried just about every diet there is. While she's managed to lose up to forty pounds in a stretch, she always gained it back, and more, because what she tried wasn't sustainable. She's been following your guidelines, and is finally learning to eat for her health."

# COMMON NUTRITION QUESTIONS

As you just read, nutrition can be ridiculously simple (and common-sense based), but you may have some looming questions.

## WHAT ABOUT SUPPLEMENTS?

Supplements are just that—they're meant to supplement healthy eating habits. No supplement can make up for poor eating habits, but they can complement good eating habits.

Know this: You're better off making it a priority to eat a wide variety of real, minimally processed foods rather than looking for the next miracle supplement. Do this and you'll likely get the nutrients and vitamins you need. Also, I am not a doctor. Don't start taking supplements without first consulting your primary-care physician, especially if you're on medication or have a medical condition.

One supplement worth considering, however, is a high-quality fish oil. Research has demonstrated several benefits from supplementing with fish oil, including reducing triglycerides and improving cardiovascular health, and it may even help with depression and reduce inflammation.[10]

But you don't have to take a fish oil supplement to get the benefits. If you eat fatty fish (e.g., salmon, herring, mackerel, sardines) each week (about two to three times), you can skip the fish oil.

Beyond that, it's a known fact that supplements are not regulated—you don't always know what you're getting in that

---

10    "Fish Oil," Examine (accessed October 27, 2017),
      *https://examine.com/supplements/fish-oil/*.

capsule or bottle. Furthermore, many supplements are poorly researched, if they've been research at all. If you want to take a supplement, like fish oil, or a health-care provider advises you to use one, get it from a reputable company that has their ingredients third-party tested, so you know what you're getting.

Ignore the sensationalized headlines about the latest fat-burning supplement that will melt fat at a rapid rate and other too-good-to-be-true promises. Save your money, and stick to the fewest things that have been proven to work. Better yet, spend it on your favorite minimally processed foods.

## DO I NEED PROTEIN POWDER?

Protein powder is excellent for convenience. Eat real, minimally processed protein sources when possible, because you'll also get vitamins and minerals in addition to the needed protein. But if you find it difficult to get plenty of protein, or you don't eat much meat or animal sources of protein, then protein powder is helpful.

Whey protein is one of the most popular options and is an excellent source of complete protein. I personally prefer whey protein isolate (instead of concentrate). It costs a bit more than concentrate, but I find it easier on my stomach, and many of my clients have reported the same (i.e., it doesn't seem to give as many people upset stomachs or the dreaded protein farts). Try both and see which one you prefer; you may do fine with the cheaper option.

Quality matters: If you're going to buy protein powder, get it from a reputable company that gets their ingredients third-party tested.

Don't want to use animal-based protein sources? No problem. Pea, rice, and hemp proteins are good plant-based protein powder options.

If you include a good source of protein with your meals
and snacks, you likely don't need to supplement with protein
powder. That said, it is a great option for convenience because
it takes a matter of seconds to mix protein powder with water,
or put a scoop in a blender with frozen fruit, a handful of spinach, and a bit of water.

Do you need a protein shake immediately after working
out? The answer is no. You don't need to slam back a protein
shake right after a workout. (This trend started when it was
thought that nutrient timing was critical.[11]) If you eat a meal
that includes a good source of protein within a few hours after
training, you don't need a shake. But if you know it's going to
be more than approximately four hours after training before
you'll eat a meal, a shake could be a good idea to supply your
body with protein.

Another opportunity for protein shakes is if you work out
first thing in the morning and don't eat a meal prior to training, and won't eat for a couple of hours or more after training. In that case, drinking a protein shake before working out
can help aid recovery from the workout. I often train in the

---

11    Alan Albert Aragon and Brad Jon Schoenfeld, "Nutrient Timing Revisited: Is
There a Post-Exercise Anabolic Window?" Journal of the International Society of
Sports Nutrition, (January 29, 2013),
https://jissn.biomedcentral.com/articles/10.1186/1550-2783-10-5.

morning and don't like having food in my stomach, so I'll drink a protein shake about fifteen minutes before training. This is personal preference: If you like having a meal/snack before a workout, then eat one. If you can't stand having food in your stomach during a workout, then don't eat, or have a protein shake.

## FOODS THAT HATE YOU

Did I mention I'm not a doctor? If you've been advised by a health-care provider not to eat something discussed above—dairy, eggs, fish, gluten, whatever—then don't eat it. The last thing I want is for someone with food allergies or a medical condition to follow the guidelines above without consulting their doctor first.

The same goes for any food that makes you feel terrible. For example, if even having a sip of milk makes you fart with such ground-shaking force that you feel like you're going to be launched into space, then don't make milk part of your protein quotient (or get a lactose-intolerant alternative).

If there are foods you loathe, or foods that don't agree with you, no problem. Simply put, focus on the abundance of foods you can eat and enjoy, not the foods you can't. This better look familiar: the *more* mentality.

## NUMBER OF MEALS

You don't need to eat a specific number of meals each day to improve your health or alter your body composition. You've likely heard that eating multiple small meals throughout the day is best for stoking the metabolic fire. The idea behind eating more frequent, smaller meals was that it would speed up metabolism. It's a nice idea, but it's been disproven by research to be superior to, say, eating three meals per day.

Research has demonstrated that eating a specific number of meals really doesn't matter when it comes to health or weight loss.[12] What matters most is doing what you enjoy and can sustain long-term. After all, if you try to revolve your life around an impractical regimen you can't sustain long-term, what's the point in doing it? The best plan for how many meals you eat is the plan that fits your life, schedule, and preferences.

For some people, that may mean three meals a day. For others, it may mean four or five because they prefer to eat smaller meals more frequently. Some individuals work long shifts with unpredicted rest breaks, so they choose to eat larger, infrequent meals.

There is no best way when it comes to meal frequency; there is only what's best for you. What you eat is more important than when you eat.

The same goes for what times of day you choose to eat. This should be dictated by what fits your lifestyle and preferences. If you hate eating breakfast because having food in your stomach early in the morning makes you feel terrible, you can skip it. If you love eating breakfast and need it to feel energized, then you should eat it.

Revolve your eating choices primarily around minimally processed foods, get sufficient protein, eat when hungry,

---

12    F. *Bellisle*, R. *McDevitt*, and A. M. *Prentice*, "Meal Frequency and Energy Balance," The British Journal of Nutrition (April 1997), *https://www.ncbi.nlm.nih.gov/pubmed/9155494.*

deliberately eat at a mindful pace, and stop when you're satisfied, but not stuffed—those guidelines matter most and are responsible for the majority of the results you will achieve.

## WAIT…THERE REALLY AREN'T ANY PROHIBITED FOODS?

We live in a new era of prohibition. Only instead of beer
and liquor, rigid diets encourage abstinence from the bliss-
ful combination of sugar, salt, and fat. It can be junk food
like snack cakes, or even high-class treats like an éclair from
a French bakery. But just like the days of speakeasies and
bootleggers, the prohibition only makes us want these items
more. It's human nature—the moment you start assigning
guilt to something, you're going to want it. As soon as you
get it, you're going to feel guilty about it. Remember the discussion about cheat meals and dichotomous thinking from
earlier? There's a reason you're banishing the good/bad and
clean/dirty food terms from your vocabulary.

Obsessing over what we should and shouldn't eat, or labeling certain foods as "bad," is how food takes control over
our lives; it dominates our thoughts. It's just food, but we
make it into something that toys with our emotions and affects our well-being and sense of self. Food is not something
to be feared.

Some people try to neutralize the fear around food by
chanting feel-good mottos like "Food is just fuel!" Frankly, I
can't get behind that approach because I tried it: eating bland,
boiled chicken breast and unseasoned broccoli because "food
is just fuel" and who cares if it tastes good. The truth is that
we're social creatures, and food is an important part of our

lives. We must know how to eat in situations where food is more than just fuel, so we can include the foods we love into social and special occasions and enjoy them without feeling guilt or remorse after eating a piece of homemade pecan pie.

Making food off-limits is the surest way to make you want it more—most of my clients have experienced this, and you probably have too. Don't play that game with guilt and self-righteousness. That's just a big pile of negativity with food at its center.

If there's a food you enjoy, you should include it in your eating choices. You should make reasonable choices about how often you enjoy it, but the last thing you should do is attempt to banish it forever. If you like to have something sweet every day, then go ahead and have a piece of chocolate or a few bites of dessert once a day. Maybe you don't need something sweet every day, but you like ordering dessert when you visit your favorite restaurant. Then go ahead and order it.

The *Lift Like a Girl* approach to nutrition is meant to be flexible, so you can make it fit your life. Apply the guidelines above and eat mostly real, minimally processed foods most of the time, and you have plenty of wiggle room for the other foods you enjoy.

"Domino" food is a particular food that's difficult to stop eating once you start. Identify your domino foods, and have a plan to handle them. For example, if the intention of eating a few nuts from the container quickly becomes half the container, scoop out a portion into a bowl, and then put the container away so you're not tempted to keep eating. If a couple of tablespoons of peanut butter turns into a quarter cup, put peanut butter in serving-size containers that you can grab when you want it. A rule of thumb: Don't eat foods straight from the bag/container. Get out what you want, or a moderate amount, and put the rest away.

My mom is an incredible cook and frequently hosts Sunday dinners for our family. One of my favorites is homemade fried chicken and okra. I'm a Southern girl, and this is a not-to-be-missed meal. I'd crawl across a field of glass shards for a plate of it. I don't eat this special meal often, but when I do, it's guilt-free.

This wasn't always the case, however. There was a time when I'd watch the rest of my family enjoy this meal full of tasty, Southern goodness while I stuck to my virtuous meal of steamed vegetables and lean protein. If I had a bite of something fried, I'd consider it a screwup or a failure of discipline.

Now I'm more objective: It's one meal over the course of a week. One meal of fried chicken, okra, and homemade mashed potatoes isn't going to change my body overnight, just like one meal (or even an entire day) of eating baked chicken, steamed broccoli, and other such foods won't make a difference on its own, either. I enjoy that special meal with my family, and then move on.

It's not the occasional fried chicken or pizza or towering ice cream cone that affects the health and composition of our bodies. It's what we do most often, over the course of weeks and months and years. And the process is simple, enjoyable, and flexible. Eat more of the minimally processed foods you enjoy, and eat the other foods less often, but also guilt-free.

## TRUST THE PROCESS

If you're used to following rigid diets and scrutinizing everything you eat from a *"Will this help me lose fat or cause me to gain fat?"* lens, the simple guidelines in this chapter may alarm you. It may be intimidating to focus on eating for overall health, feeling great, and improving your workout performance.

And the sensationalized messages from the media and health and fitness industry aren't going anywhere. There will always be a constant barrage of conflicting information, quick-fix promises, Holy Grail diets, and other marketing tactics trying to sway your attention, and money. You have to choose to disregard it. Running the information through the *"Does this sound too crazy to be true?"* test is a good start.

While research continues to provide new insight and information, the basics will not change—they are the solid foundation upon which everything else is established. While the debate rages on about what's optimal, most agree that the foundation of any healthy diet revolves around minimally processed foods. Getting plenty of protein is important, especially for individuals who participate in strength training. Flexibility with other foods is critical not only for enjoyment, but for mental health.

Nutrition needn't be complicated. If you can focus on eating more of the foods that make you feel great, more of the foods that give you energy, more of the foods that help you recover from workouts, while enjoying your favorite not-super-healthy foods occasionally, you're not going to feel deprived.

Even the obvious nutrition principles, such as not drinking sugar-laden beverages, are not what I'd prefer to have people focus on. As soon as you say, "I'm not going to drink soda anymore," drinking soda is all you're going to think about.

Focus on the delicious foods you can consume. Think abundance. Think variety. Think *more*. Eating healthy shouldn't be a punishment. You're not depriving yourself; you're giving yourself what you need to thrive. Change is easy to sustain when it's simple, flexible, and, above all, positive.

Focus on the big, important things that matter, and don't obsess over the little ones. "Should I eat a sweet potato or a regular potato?" is a very small thing that doesn't make an appreciable difference in your overall nutrition. Choosing to spend a few minutes at night prepping a protein-rich snack to take with you to work in the morning is a big thing, one that can make a difference in how awesome you feel the next day.

Commit to consistently implementing the information provided. You'll reap numerous benefits when you immerse yourself in the process.

If you're following the guidelines in this chapter, but things don't seem to be moving in the right direction, don't panic. Record what you eat and drink for a week to see what's going on. When you have the data, look for where the simplest improvements can be made. Maybe you bring a very small, unsubstantial meal to work for lunch, and your mid-afternoon hunger leaves you snacking on stale doughnuts in the break room. You identified the problem; now create a solution: add more protein and maybe veggies or a piece of fruit to your lunch, or bring a high-protein snack to work (like Greek yogurt with your favorite fruit). Track, be objective, and come up with a pragmatic solution.

## PROGRESS STARTS FROM WHERE YOU ARE TODAY

Trusting the process begins with a realistic awareness of where you're starting from. Many women I've worked with have looked at my above-mentioned nutrition guidelines and said, "That doesn't work for me. All I eat is lean meats, vegetables, and fruit, and I can't lose weight."

If that's where you find yourself now, spend a week or two tracking everything you eat and drink. You don't have to track calories or exact measurements; just write down each item you eat or drink. (Yes, even nibbles and sips count so you can get an accurate, objective picture of what's going on.)

When people practice this exercise, they sometimes realize that they were slanting the truth. They see that while they were eating lean meats, fruits, and veggies, they were also going out for a twenty-ounce café mocha a few times a week, or visiting the office candy bowl at work several times a day.

If the food journal revelations are unexpected, it doesn't make you bad, and you shouldn't feel guilty. This exercise is meant to bring awareness of how you eat, what you eat, when you eat, and maybe even why you eat (e.g., boredom). This insight is often all that's needed to make small changes that yield the biggest results. You can see what's really going on and come up with a plan of action to implement going forward.

Another element of awareness is knowing which foods are really your favorite. For example, would you rather have the stale, store-bought cookies at work, or wait until you get home to make your favorite cookies from scratch and enjoy one warm from the oven? No contest, right?

Become more powerful over the choices you make. If the only reason you'd eat the break-room cookie is because it's there, then you're not missing out on anything by walking away from it. Save that moment for a food you can enjoy the hell out of, and walk away satisfied.

Eating not-so-healthy foods in moderation is a good goal. That means you'll have to say no to certain foods occasionally—for example, not eating the doughnuts at work if you know you'd prefer to go out for your favorite ice cream. This is not saying you *can't* have a doughnut. You're simply choosing to pass on this opportunity because you'd rather eat something you really enjoy later.

## WHEN TO MAKE ONE SMALL CHANGE AT A TIME

Some people may be able to start practicing the nutrition guidelines from day one. They may instantly be able to make real-food meals and snacks, get plenty of protein each time they eat, and successfully identify physical hunger and stop eating once satisfied.

But it could be more challenging for others, especially those who are used to relying on the convenience of processed foods, fast food, and other less-than-ideal choices (or have followed rigid meal plans). If the idea of waking up tomorrow and eating mostly real, minimally processed foods seems daunting, you may want to focus on making one small change at a time.

Make one change, practice it every single day until it sticks—until it becomes a habit—and then make another change.

Many diets advocate changing everything all at once, and we expect ourselves to make a quantum lifestyle leap in order to get overnight results. But those changes don't last. The yo-yo dieting roller coaster continues: You go on a diet, vow to follow it perfectly, and the moment you slip up the tiniest bit, you go off the diet completely. Then, eventually, you try the next diet and buckle yourself right back in for the ride.

To avoid this boomerang effect, especially if the guidelines provided seem a bit daunting to implement all at once, pick one small, doable thing to change at a time.

Begin by asking: What is the simplest meal you have control over? For many people, breakfast is the easiest one (unless you prefer to skip breakfast, then you could choose lunch). Since the day has just started, nothing has distracted their attention from making a great food choice. Whatever your routine used to be—grabbing a Pop-Tart, or skipping breakfast (but then succumbing to the office doughnuts or a sugar-filled latte)—begin practicing the nutrition guidelines with that meal. Make a minimally processed, protein-rich breakfast (e.g., an omelet or scrambled eggs with veggies; a smoothie made with frozen berries, a scoop of protein powder, and a handful of kale or spinach; or oatmeal with a side of Greek yogurt). Then do this every day for at least two to three weeks.

Don't overhaul anything else—just blend and drink the smoothie (or eat your omelet and sautéed veggies, or oatmeal and Greek yogurt) every day. Enjoy it, and feel good about it.

What you're doing is giving yourself one manageable task—an action—that takes you in the right direction. Two weeks later, you'll feel good physically and feel more powerful because you did what you set out to do. Then you'll be ready for the next small change. Maybe it's getting more vegetables and protein in your lunch; maybe it's replacing your mid-afternoon, caffeine-and-sugar fix with an apple and peanut butter; maybe it's swapping out sugar-laden beverages with water or tea.

Simply identify where you can make another beneficial change with your eating habits. Then, for the next two to three weeks, continue eating the real-food breakfast and implement the new change as well. After a month, you'll have successfully made two changes to your eating habits.

Those changes add up over a few months—suddenly, you realize how many habits you've not only established, but sustained. The compounding effect is a powerful, wonderful force. This is not about perfection. It's not about feeling guilty if you forget one day or overindulge. It's about taking the right actions on a consistent basis.

When I wake up, I don't think about each movement it takes to get out of bed, start my coffee maker, or put the leash on my dog. I do it all automatically, before I've even completely woken up. You don't have to put much brainpower into your current morning routine, either. You do what you do out of habit. Our brains develop habits so that they can focus on solving more pressing and uncommon problems, and making choices. Can you imagine if we had to consciously think about every tiny maneuver we completed in our day? We'd be exhausted before we got out the door.

We can't erase habits; we can only replace them. That's the goal of the nutrition guidelines in *Lift Like a Girl*. You're not trying to erase your habit of drinking soda or eating past the point of being comfortably full. You're replacing it with another habit that makes you feel better and moves you in the direction you want to go.

An interesting fact about creating new, empowering habits is that they beget other habits. Charles Duhigg explains in *The Power of Habit* that when people start improving their eating habits, for example, they start becoming more physically active without planning to. Over time, they also start taking better care of their finances and performing better at work. Good habits have a way of building momentum and giving you the confidence to continue to become more powerful, happier, more responsible, and more awesome in all areas of your life.

## MAKE IT EASY FOR YOURSELF

While good habits make more good habits easier to develop, setting it all in motion is the most crucial part. That's why it's essential to set yourself up for success early on. In our busy lives, convenience reigns supreme. Add the brain's natural resistance to change, and you've got a situation that benefits from making your new choices as simple, and easy, as possible.

To give you an example, I realized recently I wasn't eating as many vegetables as I used to. It wasn't because I didn't like them, but because I got sick and tired of washing, chopping, and cleaning up the dishes to prepare vegetables with my meals. I objectively identified the issue: I'm not eating as many veggies as I'd like to.

I could have forced myself to get back into the chopping habit, but I would rather spend that time elsewhere. Instead, I came up with a simple remedy. I bought containers of mixed greens for salads and bags of frozen, chopped vegetables that I can microwave and serve. People can argue that microwaving frozen veggies isn't ideal and that we should all be growing our own food with homemade compost. But it's not about what's ideal—it's about what's practical. Some people will have to choose between frozen vegetables and no vegetables because they're busy, or else they will turn to the most convenient option.

Simple tip to eat more veggies: Eat a dark green, leafy salad daily. Look for spinach or spring mixes for a variety of dark greens. Look through the options to find the best price; usually the larger containers are much cheaper. My local grocer sells sixteen-ounce containers of spinach mixes for less than five dollars, and it provides about five days' worth of salads for two people. You can also add chopped cucumbers, mushrooms, peppers, onions, and tomatoes if you like those too. Be cognizant of your dressing: don't douse the salad in a high-calorie dressing. I like Greek yogurt dressing, but a bit of olive oil and lemon juice plus salt and pepper is good too. Try a few options to see what you like best.

Some people get too obsessive with healthy eating. I've been the lucky recipient of dissertation-length emails from people telling me I'm going to die because I'm heating up food in the microwave, in a plastic bag, and how dare I have the gall to call myself a fitness coach. This is one of the problems plaguing health and fitness: a constant obsession over the minute details, instead of focusing on the big picture.

I'd rather people take the simplest step than not change at all because they don't want to take the time to prepare broccoli the right way. If I see someone making the choice between eating microwaved broccoli or no broccoli, I'm going to cheer them every step of the way toward the microwave.

It's about making positive change as simple as possible. Let's calm the hell down, shall we?

Making it simple for yourself requires a little planning.

First, you may need to try a few different options to figure out what you like; maybe learn new ways to cook your real-food ingredients. An extremely useful trick is to establish a few staple meals: go-to meals or snacks that are quick and easy to prepare. It's okay to be boring—if I eat breakfast at home, I rotate between two options (the smoothie mentioned earlier and oatmeal with a chopped banana, a spoonful of peanut butter, and a scoop of unflavored protein powder).

Come up with at least a couple of meals you enjoy for breakfast, lunch, and dinner. That way, for example, if you're exhausted after a long day, you don't have to put brainpower into figuring out what's for dinner. All you need is to have a few basic foods around that are quick to put together that fulfill the guidelines—real foods, plenty of protein, fruits, and vegetables—and that you enjoy.

Be sure to keep easy-to-grab, tasty, minimally processed foods on hand when you need a quick meal or snack. If you're exhausted or famished, convenience will win out over making the best choice. Set yourself up for success by surrounding yourself with real, wholesome, nutritious foods.

There are numerous tools you can use that make eating well an easier endeavor. The slow cooker is one of my personal favorites. Simply toss the ingredients into the pot, push a button, walk away, and come home to a great meal (chili is a personal favorite and is packed with lean meat, beans, tomatoes, green peppers, onion, and spices). There are myriad recipes online and in cookbooks for slow-cooker meals, one-pot meals, and other time-saving meals as well. Try some new ones (you never know what new real foods you'll love), and save your favorites.

If preparing and cooking real-food meals is new to you, expect a learning curve. But stick with it. Once you establish this skill, it will serve you forever.

## EATING TO BECOME AWESOME

A client who was a recovering chronic dieter and who analyzed every piece of food by how it would affect her physical appearance shared an amazing experience with me. One day at work, she sat down to eat lunch at her desk: some roasted chicken, a sweet potato, a salad—a real-food meal with plenty of protein and her favorite veggies. A female coworker walked by her desk and commented, "Oh, that looks really healthy. Are you trying to lose weight?"

My client said she paused for a second, then answered, "Nope. I'm eating this to become more awesome."

That's a prime example of a powerful mindset shift. That is an amazing reason to eat real foods. People see a woman eating healthily and assume she's watching her weight—when they find out she's trying to boost her deadlift, their minds are blown.

She went on to say that her coworker stared inquisitively for a moment after hearing that response. She probably never heard another woman say anything like that before. But perhaps it stuck with her—perhaps it helped her reevaluate her own attitude toward food and her body, in a positive way.

It's time we start looking at food differently—something that's good for us, something that's meant to be enjoyable, something we can use to become as awesome as we want to be. And, yes, something to help us build a bigger deadlift.

# IT SEEMS TOO SIMPLE

There will be women who read the simple guidelines in this chapter and don't know what to do with them. If you're reading this and thinking, "Wait, that's it?" the answer is yes. That is it. And you're welcome.

If more rules, more detailed information was the answer, you would already have the results you wanted. That's what diets are by nature—a list of rigid, complicated dos and don'ts, all with a huge amount of highly detailed information to support it that make us neurotic about what we buy at the grocery and order at our favorite restaurant. It's what turns eating into a stressful challenge requiring a calculator and spreadsheet, not an enjoyable experience.

In today's information-glutted world, more information can often be detrimental to your nutrition. It creates confusion, which leads to inaction because you're wondering what's best; what's right. You scrutinize everything, comparing one rule against another.

But it can be simple, if we apply a little common sense, and are consistent with our efforts. If you strip everything down to its simplest form, you'll find it's easy to answer the question: What are the fewest things I have to do that are going to get me the majority of the results I desire?

Once you answer that question, it's a matter of application. If we're honest, that's really the challenging part. We can obsess over which rules to follow, but the challenge is committing to a change and sticking with it. It takes effort to buy real foods and pass by the tempting treats and processed, convenience foods. It takes effort to consciously pass on all the food that's offered to us at the workplace and choose instead to eat something you truly enjoy at a different time. There's a learning curve to discover new foods you enjoy and how best to prepare them. It takes time and practice to detect physical hunger and to become proficient with stopping once you're comfortably satisfied.

 Life is really simple, but we insist on making it complicated.

—*Confucius*

And, depending on your environment, you may be surrounded by people who scoff at your efforts to adopt healthy eating habits. You may be the only one in your group who orders a salad and asks for half of your entrée to be boxed up so you can take it home. You may have some challenges ahead of you. And that's okay. Acknowledge them, accept them, and plan for them.

You must be patient and know there may be a learning curve depending on your personal starting point. Don't force yourself to change everything overnight. Commit to practicing one new change at a time if needed. And then make another one. Slowly over time, you'll find your whole life transitioning into better health.

But you must be consistent. Make the changes today, tomorrow, next week, next month, next year. Master the basics. Make them habits. Most importantly, make them enjoyable habits.

You wouldn't take piano lessons for a month and then perform in a concert. You must practice the basics consistently to make discernible progress. More information isn't the answer. You know what you need to know. You just need to do it.

And, eventually, these actions will become habits—something you just do without having to put much thought into it. That's where the magic lies, and you get there one day at a time.

## HELPFUL NUTRITION TIPS

Nutrition is arguably the most difficult part of building, and sustaining, a healthy lifestyle. The information in this chapter simplified the process, and the following tips will help to further customize the guidelines to your lifestyle and preferences.

### TIP 1: DON'T FALL INTO THE ALL-OR-NOTHING TRAP.

We've discussed how most diets encourage an all-or-nothing mindset: either you do the diet perfectly without deviation, or you go off it completely and eat with reckless abandon. It may be tempting to view the real-food guideline and say, "Well, if eating real, minimally processed foods 85 percent of the time is good, then I'll get even better results if I eat those foods 100 percent of the time."

There are some people who love, and thrive from, eating real foods close to 100 percent of the time; if that's you, then go ahead. But most people have foods they enjoy that are processed, or just not super healthy (candy, baked goods, fries, etc.). Do not attempt to force yourself to abstain from any foods or food groups—thus turning the flexible guidelines into rigid rules—because you think it will lead to faster results; that's setting yourself up for failure. Follow the real-food guideline most of the time (80 percent to 90 percent) and you can easily include your favorite foods without issue, or guilt. Remember, we're not after perfection. We're after consistency with a sustainable approach.

## TIP 2: MAKE ROOM FOR FOODS YOU ENJOY THE MOST.

Maybe you like having a glass of wine with your dinner. Perhaps you love a certain candy bar. If you enjoy these foods, you must make room for them in your eating habits. If you eat real, protein-rich foods and snacks, you can include a glass of wine at night with your dinner. If you and your family visit the local bakery on Saturday morning for their special cinnamon rolls, have one guilt-free, and eat real foods for the remainder of your meals that day.

## TIP 3: DON'T FORCE YOURSELF TO EAT FOODS YOU DISLIKE.

A common complaint from some people is, "I can't eat healthy because I hate healthy foods." This is not a valid excuse. There are foods I don't like either, like beets. It doesn't matter how they're prepared, I always think they taste like dirt (you can call it an earthy taste all you want, but I feel like I just licked a freshly tilled garden). People can tout how healthy beets are, but I don't care. I hate them, so I won't eat them.

The point is that it doesn't matter what foods you hate, because there's an abundance of other foods to choose from. Focus on eating more of the real, minimally processed foods you do enjoy, and consider trying new ones. You never know when you'll discover a new favorite.

Wondering if you should do a detox or cleanse to jumpstart a healthy lifestyle? No. These gimmicks[13] promise fast

---

13   "Detoxes: An Undefined Scam," Examine (accessed October 28, 2017), *https://examine.com/nutrition/detoxes-an-undefined-scam/.*

weight loss and improved health, but they're nonsense. You have a built-in detoxing system—namely, your kidneys and liver. The best thing you can do is start establishing habits that revolve around eating mostly minimally processed foods, managing stress, getting enough sleep, and strength training regularly.

## TIP 4: MAKE HEALTHIER VERSIONS OF YOUR FAVORITE FOODS, BUT ALSO, DON'T.

If there's a certain food you want to enjoy frequently, making a healthier, real-food, nutrient-dense version of that food can be a great idea. For example, if you love fries, but know it's not a great idea to eat them every day, you can make baked fries. Cut potatoes into wedges, toss to coat in a little olive oil, sprinkle with salt and pepper, then bake for twenty to thirty minutes in a four-hundred-degree oven, flipping once halfway through. This works great with sweet potatoes too.

You can do the same thing with any other type of food as well. This way you can enjoy a familiar food frequently while ensuring that you eat mostly real, minimally processed foods.

But you shouldn't always make healthier versions of certain foods or recipes. Let's be blunt: Not every food can be made healthier and actually taste good. For example, you may be perfectly happy eating a cauliflower-crust pizza topped with a skimpy amount of low-fat cheese and sprinkled with veggies. To me, that is an abomination, undeserving of the title "pizza." When I eat pizza, it's a pizza: it has cheese, a gluten-filled crust, and generous toppings. Same thing with ice cream. Don't give me some low-fat, lower-calorie, healthier option. Nothing tastes as good as sugar-filled, full-fat ice cream.

Some foods can be made healthier and still be enjoyable. When possible, this is a good option, especially for foods you like to eat frequently. But for your favorite foods that have no good substitute and the mere thought of trying to "healthify" it insults you, enjoy them on occasion.

And, let's face it, have you tried to make a healthier version of a favorite meal or dessert that just didn't do the trick? You ended up eating more of it than you would have if you just had a reasonable amount of the real thing because: (a) you did the typical "it's healthy so I can eat a ton of it" justification, and (b) it didn't really satisfy your taste buds so you ended up eating other foods too.

One more note: Just because a recipe or product claims to be healthier than its competition doesn't always mean it really is. Oftentimes, it has the same amount of calories as the real thing it's trying to replace. And, sometimes, it even has more. Don't be fooled by labels or empty promises.

### TIP 5: SOME DAYS YOU'LL PRACTICE THE GUIDELINES BETTER THAN OTHERS—LEARN WHAT YOU CAN.

Some days you'll eat mostly real foods, get plenty of protein, and work in your other favorite, not-super-healthy foods easily. Some days, however, you may overeat and rely on heavily processed foods.

This is life, and some days are better than others. Always learn what you can. Days you follow the guidelines well, find out why that is. Maybe you had the house stocked with plenty of real foods and quick-to-prepare meals. Maybe you packed a delicious, protein-filled lunch. Find out why you were successful, and replicate it.

Likewise, on days when everything seems to have gone wrong, find out why. Perhaps you ate more of the foods you would rather eat less of, and you were overcome with guilt, so you kept making less-than-ideal food choices for the entire day. Take an objective look, and come up with a simple, pragmatic solution.

## TIP 6: MAKE THIS AS EASY AS POSSIBLE.

If you want to eat mostly real foods and plenty of protein, you need to surround yourself with real foods, and plenty of protein options. Do whatever you need to stay on track. Prep some tasty meals, buy protein-rich foods to snack on, divide "domino" foods into individual serving sizes to remove temptation. Keep fruits, nuts, protein powder, Greek yogurt, or whatever you prefer at work so you have snack options and don't succumb to the tempting call of the vending machine at two in the afternoon. You must ask yourself: What do I need to do to stay on track? How can I make this easier? Then do it.

## TIP 7: KNOW YOUR PERSONALITY, AND SET YOURSELF UP FOR SUCCESS.

Everyone is different. Some people can keep a carton of ice cream in the freezer and not be tempted on a daily basis to eat it. For others, having ice cream or other desserts in the house is a constant temptation. If it's around, they're likely to eat it until it's gone. If having your favorite treats around is a relentless test of willpower, then don't keep them in the house. Instead, when you really want a dessert or chips or whatever the food may be, go out and buy a single serving size. This way you can enjoy it, and there will be no lingering temptation to get more.

Perhaps you're the type of individual who likes having a little something sweet every day. Maybe you can eat a couple of pieces of chocolate and be satisfied without raiding the cabinets to get more. Know your personality; set yourself up to be successful.

## TIP 8: THE BEST THING YOU CAN DO IS START TODAY. RIGHT NOW.

The sooner you start practicing the nutrition guidelines, the closer you'll be to forming sustainable habits. To make sure you're moving in the right direction, consider keeping a food journal. Record what you eat and drink (the items, not the calories; e.g., two-egg omelet with sautéed veggies, twenty-ounce coffee, etc.) so you can objectively see what's happening—you don't have to rely on your memory, nor can you delude yourself from the truth.

It's not uncommon for people to swear they're following the guidelines, but rant about how their body hasn't changed. More often than not, they're not following the guidelines, and the food journal reveals this. Record what's going on for at least a week: replicate successes, and come up with a plan to handle circumstances that need attention.

## TIP 9: SAVE MONEY WHEN AND WHERE YOU CAN.

Eating real, minimally processed foods needn't be expensive. Take advantage of sales, and buy in-season produce. Look for meat that's on sale, and freeze what you don't use right away. Take advantage of bulk sales for items you'll use regularly.

Want more nutrition information? Have questions about how much protein you should eat, or how much to eat for losing fat or building muscle? Grab the free resource guide at *www.niashanks.com/book-resource-guide/*.

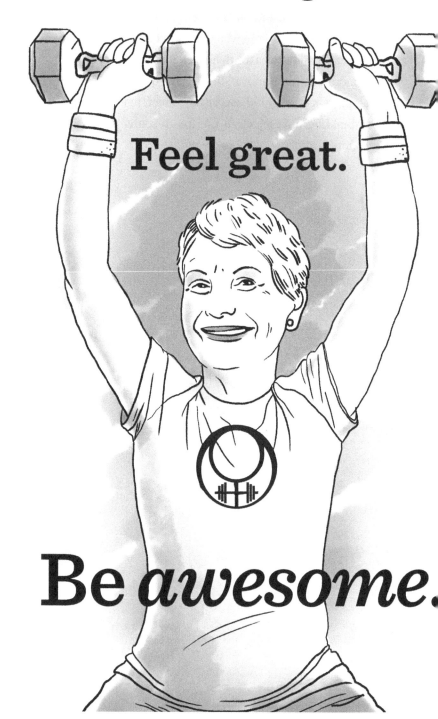

# CHAPTER 4
# The Strength Training Programs

- Decreases risk of developing metabolic syndrome
- Reduces blood pressure
- Increases bone mineral density
- Improves cognition
- Improves sleep quality
- Improves body image and confidence
- Increases strength
- Enhances performance in tasks of daily living
- May help manage and alleviate pain
- Makes you less prone to injury
- Improves balance, coordination, flexibility, and speed
- And, of course, builds muscle and aids in body fat loss

These are some of the benefits that can be attributed to a single activity: strength training. And more benefits are being researched and discovered today, thanks to the popularity of lifting weights.

So, why should women strength train?

A better question, perhaps, is why the heck wouldn't they? Strength training is a single activity that positively affects numerous other qualities. It's beautiful how efficient it is. If one activity that doesn't require a large devotion of time can provide a plethora of benefits, why wouldn't you do it?

It's worth noting that for some people, strength training close to bedtime can energize them, so it's harder to fall asleep. If this is you, don't train too close to bedtime.

But wait, there's more. Along with the external and internal benefits to physical health, strength training provides the psychological benefits we've already discussed—improving your confidence, making tasks of daily life easier, and making you feel like a capable badass no matter where you are or what you're doing.

Strength training can have a dramatic effect on your life—getting stronger means discovering all that your body is able to do. Yes, it will help you burn fat, build muscle (i.e., get toned), and provide all the aesthetic benefits. But those rewards are trifles compared to the long-term rewards of feeling empowered, confident, and capable.

Did you know strength training complements other physical activities? If you compete in running races, biking, and literally any other physical activity, increasing your physical strength will improve your performance in those activities.

Of course, there are some women who (at least initially) will proclaim not to care about feeling empowered. They just want to look better in a swimsuit or favorite pair of jeans. If that's your goal, the strength training programs will get you there. Don't be surprised, however, when you experience the other phenomenal benefits that come along with that goal.

Maybe best of all, you'll be astonished when you discover how much you enjoy the process. Even women who normally hate taking the time to work out end up looking forward to, and enjoying, the *Lift Like a Girl* strength training program, precisely because it doesn't require hours out of their week or going through a dozen or more different exercises in one session.

## LIFT LIKE A GIRL IN REAL LIFE

"It took me two weeks to find the courage to break free of my grueling and tedious sixty-minute, five times a week weight training sessions. After two weeks, I'm loving the energy I have post-workout, and not stressing about squeezing in five long sessions. AND I'm still getting stronger."

Strength training delivers myriad benefits in a safe, proven, single approach. What's not to love about that?

## WILL I GET BULKY?

I have no idea.

Not the answer you expected? I can't say, "No," because what's considered bulky is entirely subjective. For example, I don't classify myself as bulky, but some women do. What one woman may consider bulky is not enough bulk to another. The real solution here is to (a) not comment on other women's bodies; (b) not care about what other people think of your body; and (c) learn to embrace words like *grow*, *strong*, and, yes, even *muscle*, and to abolish the irrational fear that lifting weights will do anything but provide incredibly positive and rewarding results.

This idea that as soon as a woman starts lifting weights she's going to magically and quickly expand and grow dramatically is absolute nonsense. This is perpetuated by the idea that one should lose fat before building muscle. This misinformation has been used to encourage women to do cardio to lose fat, and then later, once they've lost body fat, start lifting (very light) weights. It also contributes to the language marketers use to sell gimmicky workout tools made just for women that promise to tone and build long and lean muscles that don't bulk you up. This is utter rubbish.

> What is meant by the word *tone* (i.e., "I don't want to bulk up, I just want to tone") is what happens when you build muscle and lose body fat. That is what creates the toned look, and strength training is the tool for the job.

Let's clear up any confusion: There's a difference between weight loss and fat loss. Hours and hours of cardio will help you lose fat, but it also has the potential to make you lose muscle. So while you may technically weigh less, you aren't going to have a toned appearance.

Strength training is a tool that will allow you to build a healthy, proportionate amount of muscle mass for your body. Furthermore, strength training aides in fat loss, so it's a win-win. That's the beauty of a proper progressive strength training program—it's the one tool that lets you change the shape and appearance of your body in a dramatic fashion while also contributing to better overall health.

Let's commit to no longer having the "I don't want to get bulky" discussions around weight lifting. Let's stop allowing myths and nonsense to make us afraid of getting strong, building muscle, and become more. When you follow sound nutrition guidelines (from chapter 3) and regularly strength train with the goal of getting stronger, your body will respond by losing fat and building muscle. This will dramatically affect how you feel, look, and perform. You'll just have to experience it for yourself.

Strength training is the one tool that can radically change the shape of your body while improving your overall health. Women routinely comment how their breasts seem to get bigger, or at least perkier from strength training (even women who breast-fed multiple children). Women also report filling out their jeans because their butt is more round, full, and perky. Bottom line, even from an appearance-based perspective, building muscle is a good thing.

# IT'S OKAY WHEN YOUR GOALS CHANGE

Our goals inevitably change as we get older; our lives change, and we have different experiences. A woman in her twenties may want to feel more confident in her clothes. A woman in her forties may be interested in increasing her strength and stamina so she can keep up with her kids. A woman in her seventies may want to get stronger so she can maintain her independence. Whereas nothing but a desire to look better may have got a woman working out at first, wanting to feel great, be strong, and have energy to do the activities she loves outside the gym is what may keep her working out long-term.

My mom, also a personal trainer, specializes in training senior citizens. One of her clients has been training with her for sixteen years, and this client is now in her early nineties. This woman isn't interested in how she looks in a swimsuit; she wants to be able to travel on her own, get in and out of the bathtub, get up from her chair and answer the door, and climb in and out of her car without needing assistance. Her goal with exercise is to maintain her independence.

This is an example of the importance of making strength training part of your life right now. The point is to build strength and muscle and bone, and to make it part of your life so you keep doing it as you age. The sooner you establish the habit of strength training, the better off you'll be. And, no, it's never too late, regardless of whether you're forty or eighty-seven.

That's another wonderful fact about strength training—it doesn't discriminate. It doesn't matter how old you are or what limitations you have—everybody can strength train to some degree, and make real, noticeable progress toward their individual goals. Even with injuries or physical limitations, there's always something you can do. There's always somewhere you can improve. That's why strength training is awesome. There's no reason not to do it. It's an activity that can improve every person, in multiple ways.

## IS STRENGTH TRAINING SAFE?

The short answer is yes. As long as you learn and use proper form, use a weight you can control at all times, and apply proper safety measures, it's proven to be a safe activity.

Frequently, people who decide to start strength training go into a gym, choose weights they think they can handle, and start moving them up and down without thinking about what they're doing. Suddenly, mid-squat, their knees are sending up alarm signals. These people will limp home and say, "Squats are bad for my knees" or "Strength training isn't safe."

Unfortunately, there are doctors and even physical therapists who will confirm this misconception. If a patient comes in with a sore muscle or injury and says it happened while they were lifting weights, some doctors will advise against doing it ever again.

I'm not telling you to disregard your doctor's advice. In particular, if you have a musculoskeletal injury, you should do what your physical therapist says. I am, however, saying that sometimes it's beneficial to seek a second opinion. Doctors don't take a course on strength training in medical school, and many physical therapists don't, either. Thankfully, there's a growing field of medical professionals who are avid strength trainees themselves, so they know the benefits of the activity and encourage their patients to strength train. (Many of these doctors even use strength training to treat pain, movement, and health conditions.)

I recommend that everyone tries to work with a medical provider who is knowledgeable about strength training. That way, if you experience an injury, your doctor/physical therapist can not only help you heal, but will create a plan to work within your limitations so you can, over time, do the activities you want to do.

Limitations aside, the key to safety in strength training is executing the movements correctly. If you want to reap the benefits of strength training, commit at the beginning to learn proper form. It's much easier to take a little longer to learn correct form in the beginning, than to develop bad habits that must be corrected later.

Some of the exercises used in the program require certain safety precautions. It's a sad fact that a lot of accidents happen every year because people didn't have a spotter, or didn't use safety bars when bench pressing. These accidents are completely preventable.

Respect what you're doing, while you're doing it. If you have a barbell on your back and squat down, your mind should be focused on one thing: performing that rep. Focus intently on what you're doing and the proper cues for that lift, and you'll get the most benefit out of the movement, safely.

A rule of thumb when strength training is to focus on the movements. Concentrate completely on every rep of every set. Make sure you're following the coaching cues (provided with the demonstration photos of each exercise).

Safety tip: The last rep of a set should look identical to the first. The exception: The speed may be a bit slower (meaning, the last rep of a squat may come up a bit slower than the first, due to fatigue). Don't sacrifice proper exercise form to complete an extra rep, or to use more weight. Don't attempt a rep that you're not confident you can complete with good form.

## WILL I, OR WON'T I, LOSE WEIGHT?

Muscle is more dense than fat: Ten pounds of muscle take up less space than ten pounds of fat. This is why a woman can strength train for several months and "only" drop five pounds of bodyweight, but look radically different. While she lost fifteen pounds of fat, she built ten pounds of muscle. Even though the scale shows "just" a five-pound loss, a change in body composition makes a tremendous visual difference.

### LIFT LIKE A GIRL IN REAL LIFE

"I've been blown away by the way my body has changed in the last seven weeks, and I'm excited to see how it will morph in the next fifteen. You are an absolute legend! I love your 'no frills' approach to weight training. I am HOOKED."

A woman with quite a bit of excess body fat will experience a bigger drop on the scale, even though she also built muscle. Someone who isn't significantly overweight when they start strength training won't see as large of a difference on the scale. As mentioned in chapter 1, this tends to discourage some women. They may notice dramatic differences in how they feel, how their body looks, and even how their clothes fit. But then they step on the scale and don't see the huge drop they were expecting.

It can be challenging to disconnect from the "less equals better" mentality—the scale does not tell the whole story. This is why I tell women to put away the scale if the number they see tends to elicit an emotional response—to stop making that the indicator of success.

Depending on your starting point, the scale may not change much, but you absolutely will look and feel different.

> If you're used to relying on the bathroom scale to indicate your success, or lack thereof, try this: Forget about trying to make the number on the scale go down. Commit to making the weight on the barbell go up.

You can't fake being strong, and you can't conceal weakness. If daily activities like climbing stairs or picking up your kid are a struggle, it affects your entire life.

That's why becoming strong affects your entire life in an equally significant way. It's such an exciting experience when what you're doing in the gym spills over into real life, and truly improves every part of it. Oftentimes, your newly gained strength affects daily life in ways you never considered. You'll find yourself exclaiming, "Wow! This used to make me winded, and here I am tossing these things around like they're feather pillows." It really helps you see what your body is capable of doing, and leaves you asking, "What else can I do?"

## LIFT LIKE A GIRL IN REAL LIFE

"I finally back-squatted a barbell loaded with the equivalent of my bodyweight! It finally clicked: the whole idea of training for *performance*, getting stronger, and not relying so heavily on numbers (whether they be scale numbers, calories burned or consumed, macronutrient percentages, etc.)."

This isn't to downplay the achievements in the gym. It's amazing for women when they discover that, yes, they absolutely can do perfect traditional push-ups. They can get to the point where they're doing unassisted chin-ups. They can reach an awesome milestone such as deadlifting one and a half times their bodyweight, and often much more.

Being stronger in the gym gives you a push to go out and try activities you've always wanted to do, but weren't sure if you could. The mental transformation that occurs once you're squatting the equivalent of your bodyweight makes it a lot easier to stare down something that used to intimidate you and think, "Hell yeah, I can do that."

So let's revisit the original question: Why should women strength train?

Look at it this way: If there was one activity you could do that would provide a long list of incredible benefits, why wouldn't you do it? If this one activity can help you lose fat;

build muscle; improve your bone mineral density, balance, and coordination; and so much more, while possibly making you smarter and lifting your boobs...why wouldn't you give it a try?

## BEGINNING IS THE BEST PART

It's important to remember that strength training is an acquired skill. There are some fundamentals to learn in the beginning that will provide the foundation for quicker progress. Exercises that can be learned quickly were specifically chosen for Phase 1 to shorten the learning curve. If you feel intimidated at first, know that taking it slower and easier is the best way to go.

If anything, you should be excited because—and you may not expect this—being a beginner is awesome. It's the time you can make the quickest progress and initial strength gains. The first several months of strength training is when linear progression is at its peak, simply because your body isn't accustomed to the activity and you haven't expressed your strength potential. Every week you're able to add more weight, do more reps, kick more ass. Once you get past the brief learning curve to establish proper form for the exercises, you'll progress quickly. And it's dang fun.

This is also the peak time you'll be able to lose fat and build muscle simultaneously, thus changing your body composition greatly.

As you get stronger, though, linear progression slows down. Instead of adding five pounds to the bar, you may have to add two and a half, and then only one pound for certain exercises. This is when strength training brings in another learned benefit, patience. This is when you must recommit to the process, and realize nothing progresses in a linear fashion forever. Whereas gains came quickly in the beginning, later you'll have to work a little harder for a lot less. You must embrace the process and apply a hefty dose of patience and perseverance. This is something you won't experience until a few months into the Phase 2 program, once you've built a solid strength foundation.

Strength training provides mental discipline. You must commit to learning proper form; you must show up and put in the work. When progress slows down, you must be patient and immerse yourself in the process. Whether your goal is to bust out a flawless set of push-ups, achieve a bodyweight chin-up, or squat your bodyweight for reps, you must persevere. These goals are all doable, and some may take longer than others to achieve. But stick with it. This mental discipline in the gym will spill over into everyday life, often in ways you didn't expect.

Enjoy the quick initial progress, and take advantage of it. Then when it slows down, celebrate that you made it to that point. Then keep going. Keep progressing.

## WHAT MAKES THE BIGGEST DIFFERENCE

Reaping the greatest benefits from strength training means doing what matters most: using the best exercises, using appropriate volume (combination of sets and reps), training the movements frequently, improving performance, and being consistent. The *Lift Like a Girl* programs are designed with these ruling principles.

The best exercises are specific movements that are the most efficient—they provide the greatest value for your time and effort. They train a lot of muscle mass through an appropriate range of motion, improve strength, build muscle and bone, and improve other qualities like coordination, balance, and stability. The exercises used in the programs are functional in the best possible sense of the word. Just think about what you do on a daily basis: you squat (squat movement pattern) to get in and out of a chair, you pick things up off the floor (deadlift movement), you put items over your head onto a shelf/in a cabinet (overhead press movement).

Wondering what equipment you'll need for the strength training programs? The *Lift Like a Girl* workouts use dumbbells, barbells, a chin-up bar, a power rack, and a weight bench.

Some gyms nowadays have Smith machines in lieu of free weight barbells. If that's your only option, use it; you must make do with what's available. But a barbell is preferred and should be used if possible, and it is used often in Phase 2.

It may be that your gym doesn't have some of the equipment used in the workouts. Or you may encounter an exercise you can't perform, due to physical limitations. You can use appropriate alternatives with whatever equipment is available (or to work around any physical limitations or injuries), which you can get in the free resource guide at *www.niashanks.com/book-resource-guide/.*

Combine all those traits, and you'll quickly understand why a squat (goblet squat in Phase 1, barbell squat in Phase 2) is used in the *Lift Like a Girl* programs instead of a leg press, or a machine that mimics the squatting motion. A squat, compared to a leg press, not only trains your legs (as well as glutes, abs, and lower back), but it also builds coordination and balance. This isn't to say that the leg press is a bad exercise; the squat is simply more efficient, and arguably more functional. Remember, the goal with the workout programs isn't just to get strong, but to improve as many other qualities as possible in the most efficient way.

The programs are designed with specific exercises to train the entire body effectively, and they have progressive loading potential (meaning an opportunity to do more reps, add more weight). After all, I'm assuming you have a life outside of the gym. In addition to improving your health and strength, you want to be able to spend time with your family and friends, pursue other interests and hobbies, and live your life more fully.

To achieve the greatest results while spending only as much time in the gym as you have to, you must use the best exercises to accomplish that goal. But don't worry—I've got the exercise selection covered for you.

Once you have the best exercises, your job is to improve your performance in every workout. Strength training results are all about requiring your body to adapt. If you're not presenting your body with a new challenge each time, it has no reason to build muscle and bone.

That's why getting stronger is a worthwhile goal—it's

both measurable and fun. It's also why you'll be using heavier weights and performing lower rep sets—this is better for building strength than light weights and high reps. If you squatted ninety-five pounds last week for five reps, doing one hundred pounds for five reps this week means you improved your performance. The data is there. You can't deny it. We'll get into how to push yourself safely when we go through the workouts.

Maximum effectiveness is one side of efficiency; the other side is minimum time spent. There are two strength training programs in this book, and each program has two workouts, with three exercises per workout. This may come as a shock to those who are used to doing four times as many exercises when they visit the gym, including every exercise in the book to improve a specific body part. Especially if you're used to searching on Google "how to lose weight fast," it's easy to think you have to do a wide selection of exercises.

But you won't be training individual body parts in the *Lift Like a Girl* programs. You'll be training big movement patterns that work a lot of muscle at once. For example, instead of saying, "I want to work on my butt and thighs," you're going to build a bigger squat, because it works your legs, butt, and other supporting musculature as well.

If you're used to spending an hour or more at the gym, don't panic. The exercises used in this program ensure that you work the greatest muscle mass possible for maximum efficiency. I'll explain this in more detail in a moment. You must focus on putting your energy into the fewest exercises that will give you the greatest benefits.

Not convinced? Here's why it works better this way: If you only have three exercises (as opposed to ten or more), you won't be tempted to rush through the workout because you still have ten more to go. By putting complete focus and effort into each exercise, you're going to get the fullest benefit from it, and this is much easier to do with only a few exercises.

The other benefit is a gentler learning curve. Think about it: Are you going to more quickly learn proper technique with three exercises, or ten? My goal is to set you up for success. If you're trying to learn too much from the outset, there's a chance you're going to think, "I can't get this, it's too complicated. This is frustrating."

Instead, exercises you can learn quickly *and* safely have been selected, so you can start seeing progress immediately. It's about picking a few movements you're going to repeat frequently, so you get to practice proper form, seal in the correct technique, and master the movement more quickly than if you were doing dozens of exercises.

A simple example is the upper arms. Many women come to me moaning, "I hate the back of my arms. I've been doing tricep kickbacks and push-downs and all this stuff. Help me get my arms to look better."

What they don't know is that single-joint, isolation exercises (like kickbacks and push-downs) are not the best choices for improving the appearance of their arms, especially if they want to be efficient with their training. The better option is to focus on building strength with multi-joint, compound exercises (push-ups, bench presses, overhead presses). For targeting the upper arms, for example, push-ups are terrific; they challenge the triceps, but they also work the chest, anterior shoulders, stomach, and lower back from stabilizing the body. By contrast, a tricep kickback is working one muscle, and with nowhere near the amount of weight possible with a compound exercise like a push-up or barbell press (heavier loads recruit a greater percentage of muscle fibers).

Furthermore, the tricep muscles cross two joints (elbow and shoulder) and an exercise like a push-down only trains *one* of the triceps' functions, the elbow extension. A push-up, however, trains all heads of the triceps from executing elbow and shoulder extension simultaneously. You can also progress a push-up or barbell bench press (i.e., get stronger) to a much greater extent than an isolation exercise. This is why the *Lift Like a Girl* programs use compound, multi-joint exercises.

Time and time again, once a woman starts busting out flawless push-ups and achieves her first bodyweight chin-up, she has the great-looking arms she wanted. Not to mention, she's much stronger, confident, and capable in a way a tricep push-down could never deliver. This is training economy in practice.

Ready to get started? I knew you would be.

## RESPECT THE ACTIVITY

This is important, and beneficial: Make every rep count. Don't blast through the first three reps to hurry and get the set over with. Focus on what you're doing. Treat every rep in the workout, even the warm-ups, like it's the only one you get to do.

People don't understand why I stress this, until they come back after a week of diligently applying this advice. "Oh my gosh," they'll say, "I didn't realize how big of a difference that makes." You get more out of the activity if you respect it and mentally prepare for it.

This becomes even more crucial as you get stronger. If you're squatting with a barbell loaded to sixty-five pounds, you need to be focused, and this is more important when there's 150 pounds on your back. Focus intently, and respect the activity from the beginning; this way it'll be habit as you get stronger and the weights get heavier.

Your motto when training: Make every rep count.

That brings up another point. If you're new to strength training, or at least new to the exercises used in the programs, you'll have to get used to the sensation of a heavy weight on your back or in your hands. I've found it to be common that, when a woman is introduced to strength training, she *thinks* a weight is really heavy and is hesitant to add more. The feeling of having to resist a weight and balance is foreign, and even uncomfortable. While she can physically control and lift the weight, her mind may see things differently.

This is completely normal. You're capable of more than you realize, and the programs will unleash your potential. After several weeks of training, your confidence will grow, and your exercise form will be smooth and solid.

## RESPECT YOUR OWN PACE

Don't compare your strength or performance to anyone else. Respect your starting point and work at your own pace—you can't jump ahead or catch up to anyone else (or a previous version of yourself). This is *your* journey.

Everyone was a beginner at some point, including me. I didn't emerge from the womb and start busting out chin-ups, nor did I achieve a double-bodyweight deadlift in a few short months of training. I had to learn all the exercises too. It took time to get strong, and more time to get even stronger. At this point, I've been strength training close to two decades. But I didn't get to where I am by trying to match another woman's pace.

Someone who is strength training for the first time is going to have a different journey from someone who has strength training experience. Even if you're athletic and work out regularly, acknowledge your own learning curve, whatever it looks like. If it takes you twenty minutes to learn an exercise, who cares? You're in it to become more awesome on your own terms, not to fulfill some outside standard. It's important that every woman treats her journey with respect; you're not competing with anyone. Focus on doing a little better every time you repeat a workout.

> Is there a best time of day to work out? Yep, there is—whenever you'll actually do it.

You're going to get stronger, but it will be at your own pace; someone else's performance is irrelevant. Respect your journey, and the fact that you're on it. The point isn't where you start or end. The point is that you move forward, consistently.

## RESPECT YOUR BODY

If you're new to strength training, or starting back after a long layoff, don't do too much right away and risk getting brutally sore. You don't want to wake up the next day after a workout and struggle to get out of bed...and off the toilet. If needed, for the first week perform two sets (instead of the allotted four) for each exercise. If you don't get too sore, next week increase the sets to three for each exercise, and the week after you should be able to do all four work sets without a problem. This will make sense when you see the workouts.

Most women who heed this advice thank me later. In the past, they did too much too soon and ended up so sore that it negatively affected their daily tasks. Oftentimes, this caused them to hate exercise all over again, and they quit going to the gym. But once they gave themselves the freedom to move at their own pace, they felt good after working out. Sure, they still got a little sore, but it was completely manageable. This made working out empowering instead of draining, the way it's supposed to be, and it left them excited to get back and do it again.

## LIFT LIKE A GIRL IN REAL LIFE

"I cannot recall a time when I have ever been as excited about training as I am right now. I just did my workout today and yet I am so anxious to go back and work again! I can't wait to get in there and push harder and see what more I can do again and again. *Thank you so much, Nia!* Your encouragement, positivity, and awesome programs have made a *huge* impact on my whole life. I cannot thank you enough!"

# SEQUENCE OF STRENGTH TRAINING

Resist the temptation to skip this part and flip straight to the workouts. There are some important components and instructions you must follow to get the best results and stay safe. If you feel confused at any point or aren't sure what to do, revisit this section. The following information applies to Phases 1 and 2.

## GENERAL WARM-UP

The purpose of the general warm-up is to gradually increase circulation and heart rate; it increases blood flow to the muscles and lubricates joints.

> A warm-up becomes even more important during cold months. Extend your warm-up a few extra minutes.

Walk on a treadmill, ride a stationary bike, or use calisthenics like jumping jacks for about five minutes. A rule of thumb is when you've broken a light sweat, you're ready to move on to the specific warm-up.

## SPECIFIC WARM-UP

After the general warm-up you'll perform warm-up sets for all exercises. The goal is to get your body prepared for the movements, hone proper technique, get your mind focused, and prepare you to handle the heavier weights used for the work sets. The warm-up sets are also great for working on mobility.

A work set is what's listed in the workouts. For example, 4x5-7 means to perform four work sets of five to seven reps per set. Warm-up sets are *not* included in the workouts.

This is where things go to hell for a lot of people. They think, "Oh, warm-ups are just to get me ready for the rest of the workout," and then rush through it mindlessly. That is a crucial mistake.

The warm-up prepares you to get the maximum benefit out of the workout. It's as much for the mind as for the body. It sets the tone for what you're about to do. If you're about to squat one hundred pounds, and warm-up with an empty forty-five-pound barbell, perform the warm-up treating that barbell as though there are two hundred pounds on it. You're going to make sure your feet are set, your shoulder blades are together, and your back is locked in a neutral position.

**Helpful tip:** Most standard barbells weigh forty-five pounds. If you're not sure how much the ones at your gym weigh, find out. There are some barbells that weigh thirty-five pounds, and they're often best for women to start with, especially for the press and bench press in Phase 2. For the sake of example with warm-up and work sets in this book, it's assumed that an empty barbell weighs forty-five pounds.

Treat every warm-up set like it's a work set. Perform every rep deliberately, with purpose and focus. This way, once the weight is heavier, your mind and body are fully prepared.

If you feel low on energy, you feel more stiff than usual, you're training in a very cold environment, your exercise technique feels off, or your mobility feels limited, extend the warm-up. A good guide is to repeat the first warm-up set one to two more times until the movement feels better and you achieve proper range of motion.

How many warm-up sets should you do? This depends on personal preference, strength, and the exercise. You want to get ready for the work sets (what's shown in the workout programs), but don't want to accumulate much fatigue. Perform one to four warm-up sets, depending on the exercise and your preferences. Note: Older trainees, or those with a long injury history, tend to prefer more warm-up sets.

The more weight an exercise can handle, the more warm-up sets are needed. If you're going to deadlift 185 pounds for the work sets, you'll need more warm-up sets than you will for something like a dumbbell shoulder press, which you may be using ten to twenty pounds for. As you get stronger, you'll want to add another warm-up set or two.

Perform the first warm-up set with a light weight for eight to ten reps; add a little weight and do three to five more reps. Add more weight again if a third warm-up is needed or desired, and perform one to three more reps. A little personalization here is fine—some people find they feel better with a couple of extra warm-up sets, while some people find that after two to three they're ready to go. Play around and see what works best for you.

Here's a warm-up example with goblet squats (used in Phase 1). The workout calls for four sets of five to seven reps—these are the work sets. Important reminder: Warm-up sets are *not* listed in the workouts.

- Warm-up set #1: 10 x 10 (10 pounds, 10 reps)
- Warm-up set #2: 20 x 5 (20 pounds, 5 reps)
  - Work sets: 30 x 4 x 5 (30 pounds, 4 sets, 5 reps each set)

Here's an example with the deadlift, used in Phase 2. To bring this example to life, let's assume the gym is colder than usual and the first warm-up set didn't feel too great:

- Warm-up set #1: 45 x 10 (empty barbell, 10 reps)
- Warm-up set #2: 45 x 10 (repeated the first warm-up; first set didn't feel great)
- Warm-up set #3: 95 x 5 (95 pounds, 5 reps)
- Warm-up set #4: 135 x 3 (135 pounds, 3 reps)
  - Work sets: 185 x 4 x 5 (185 pounds, 4 sets, 5 reps each set)

Remember, the purpose of the warm-up sets is to hone proper technique and prepare your body and mind for the work sets. A good warm-up guideline is to increase the weight each warm-up set, while decreasing the reps performed. Start with eight to ten reps for the first warm-up set; add weight and perform three to five reps for the second warm-up; if a third warm-up is needed, add weight and perform one to three reps. Perform more warm-ups if needed or desired.

If you're unable to perform some of the exercises in the workout programs due to a lack of equipment, please see the free resource guide for appropriate alternatives at *www.niashanks.com/book-resource-guide/*.

## HOW TO WARM-UP WITH BODYWEIGHT EXERCISES?

Push-ups and inverted rows are used in Phase 1 and chin-ups in Phase 2; they need a warm-up set or two as well. To perform warm-up sets, all you'll need to do is make those exercises easier, applying the same warm-up method above. Making those exercises easier, in this case, means putting the barbell in the power rack (or Smith machine) at a higher level than you'll use for the work sets (don't worry, this is explained shortly), then lowering it for each warm-up set for push-ups and inverted rows. For chin-ups you'll need a thicker resistance band to provide greater assistance for warm-up sets.

## REST PERIODS

How long should you rest between sets of an exercise?

When starting Phase 1, the rest periods between sets of an exercise will likely be forty-five to sixty seconds. Since you're new to the activity, you won't be using much weight, so you won't need as much time to recover between sets of an exercise.

A few key strength training terms.

**Set:** A group of consecutive reps.

**Rep (i.e., repetitions):** A single, complete movement of an exercise.

Workouts consist of exercises performed for a specific number of sets and reps. For example, "Goblet squat: 4x5-7" means to perform four work sets of five to seven reps per set. (Remember, this number does *not* include warm-up sets.)

Be aware that the further you get into Phase 1, and especially Phase 2, the more rest you will need between sets, not less. That's because you'll be handling heavier weights—your muscles need more time to recover so you can put full effort into the following sets.

A couple of months into Phase 2, you may rest two to three minutes between sets of an exercise, especially those that can handle a lot of weight, like squats and deadlifts.

A good rule is that the more weight an exercise uses, the longer you'll want to rest between sets. Rest as long as needed to put full effort into the following set. If you discover your strength plummets on subsequent sets of the same exercise (for example, if you completed seven reps on set one but could only do four on the second set), you're likely not resting enough. Increase the rest period by one minute, and see if that helps.

The same guidelines apply to rest between different exercises. At the beginning of Phase 1 you may only need to rest between exercises as long as it takes to set up the equipment for the next exercise. Once you're several weeks into Phase 2, you may want to rest a couple of minutes between exercises, so you're a bit fresher for the next lift.

## THE COOL-DOWN

Once you complete a workout, don't just get in your car and drive home. Perform light activity (something as simple as walking around) for three to five minutes to bring your heart rate down.

## LIFTING TEMPO

You don't need to count how many seconds it takes to lower and lift the weight, but you should control every portion of the rep. As a general guideline, take about two seconds to perform the lowering portion of a rep (e.g., when squatting down with a goblet or barbell squat, or as you're lowering yourself down from the top of a push-up). Then, *smoothly* reverse the motion and complete the rep.

Using the squat as an example, take about two seconds to squat down to proper depth (explained later), and once you reach that depth, immediately and smoothly reverse the motion and squat back to the top, which will take about one to two seconds.

All reps should look smooth and controlled at all times.

## IF SOMETHING HURTS

Pain is typically the result of not doing an exercise correctly. If something hurts, stop what you're doing and go back to the book. Study the photos and reread the coaching cues. Then try it again, using less weight if needed, and make sure you're applying the provided cues. Usually it's a simple fix; for example, if someone says squats hurt their knees, they simply need to make sure their knees track in line with their toes when squatting.

If you're certain you're doing the exercise properly, and pain persists, stop that exercise for the day. If possible, perform an alternative exercise you can do pain-free. For example, if deadlifts just don't feel good (maybe you did a ton of yard work the day before and your back is still fatigued), swap them out for Romanian deadlifts with a light weight.

If the pain persists, go see a physical therapist, preferably one who is knowledgeable about strength training.

**Helpful tip:** Record yourself. If you're not sure you're doing something correctly, or want to make sure you are doing a movement correctly, watching yourself on video makes it easy to find out. By comparing your performance of the exercise with the photos and coaching cues in this book, you can make real-time adjustments and ensure that you're building proper technique. This is good to do occasionally to make sure your form stays solid, especially as the weights get heavier.

## HOW MUCH WEIGHT SHOULD I USE?

I can't tell you how much weight to use for every exercise; there are too many variables that go into that decision (your experience with the exercise, strength, etc.). If you're new to training, start with a weight you can easily handle to learn proper form. After a workout or two, once you're comfortable with the exercises, strive to use a weight that's challenging, but still lets you maintain proper form on all reps.

If after the first couple of weeks of training you're performing five reps with a weight you could lift ten or more times, it's not heavy enough.

As a general guideline, most exercises in the strength training programs use a five to seven rep range. Aim to use a weight you know you can handle for the high end of the rep range (seven reps in this example), but start at the low end of the rep range. Each time you repeat the workout, do a little better (as I'll explain in a moment). But it's always better to start too light because you can add weight.

## HOW LONG SHOULD IT TAKE TO COMPLETE A WORKOUT?

This will vary among individuals and between the two different strength training programs. A beginner starting out with Phase 1 may likely complete the workouts, at least for the first couple of weeks, in half an hour. Since they won't be using much weight, they won't have to rest much between sets or exercises.

As a trainee progresses in Phase 2, the workouts will take approximately one hour to complete, because they'll be handling heavier weights and need longer rest periods.

But, again, the time it takes to complete each workout will depend on how long someone performs the general warm-up, how many warm-up sets they perform, and how long they rest between exercises. Most people, however, complete the entire workout in one hour.

## HOW MANY WORKOUTS DO I PERFORM EACH WEEK?

For Phases 1 and 2, perform three workouts per week on non-consecutive days. Something like Monday, Wednesday, Friday or Tuesday, Thursday, Saturday is ideal.

Now that you know how to prepare for and perform each workout, let's get into the individual programs and their specific instructions.

## LIFT LIKE A GIRL PHASE I

There are two *Lift Like a Girl* strength training programs. Phase 1 is an introductory phase and uses exercises that are easiest to learn, while teaching you important movement patterns you'll build on in Phase 2. For example, the goblet squat (popularized by Dan John) is a great way to learn the squatting movement pattern. The Romanian deadlift teaches a movement known as a hip hinge. These movements also teach you to adopt a rigid, board-like position with your back, which is important for staying safe and building strength.

Once you've built a foundation of strength and learn proper movement patterns, Phase 2 uses exercises that allow for more strength progression, because they have a greater loading potential. For example, you'll be able to add weight more consistently with a barbell squat (in Phase 2) than you can with a goblet squat (in Phase 1).

As stated earlier, you'll perform three workouts per week on nonconsecutive days.

For most people, three workouts a week is manageable. Feel free to adapt this if it's not. You can still achieve great results with two workouts per week. Rule of thumb: Perform three when possible, but if you have a week when you can only do two, then do two! It's better than none, after all.

Giving your body a day off between workouts helps you recover, so you can put the greatest effort into the next workout. This is why it's recommended to perform the workouts on nonconsecutive days. The workouts are important, but so is recovering from them.

There are two workouts in Phase 1 that you'll rotate throughout the week—A, B, A one week, and then the next week B, A, B. The goal is to give you a high frequency of exposure with these movements, allowing you to get stronger quicker. Here's how it will look, assuming you work out on Monday, Wednesday, and Friday:

Week 1:
- Monday: Workout A
- Wednesday: Workout B
- Friday: Workout A

Week 2:
- Monday: Workout B
- Wednesday: Workout A
- Friday: Workout B

...and keep repeating.

### *LIFT LIKE A GIRL* PHASE 1 WORKOUTS

The main purpose of Phase 1 is to get accustomed to strength training and using exercises that can be learned quickly. Follow Phase 1 for a minimum of four weeks (if you're not new to strength training) or upwards of 12 weeks (if you're brand new to strength training or coming back after a long layoff). Then move on to Phase 2.

Workout A:
1. Goblet squat: 4x5-7
2. Push-up: 4x5-7
3. Inverted row: 4x5-7

Workout B:
1. Romanian deadlift (RDL): 4x5-7
2. Standing dumbbell press: 4x5-10
3. Goblet squat: 4x5-7

Is lifting heavy weights for five to seven reps safe? Isn't it safer to perform ten or more reps? Most women, if they have strength trained, are accustomed to using higher reps and lower weight. Part of the reason is the myth that light weights are better for toning and heavy weights add bulk. That's nonsense. Any rep range can build muscle with appropriate volume and muscle fatigue. Lower reps are used here because (a) they're better for building strength since they allow heavier weights to be used and recruit a greater percentage of muscle fibers, and getting strong is awesome; and (b) the argument can be made that lower reps are actually safer than higher reps—it's easier to stay focused for five reps as opposed to ten or more. Bottom line: If you use proper form and a weight you can control at all times, heavier weights are safe.

Don't worry—the entire workout is explained below. Let's go over how to correctly perform each exercise, and then you'll see how to perform each workout and how to improve your performance over time.

## GOBLET SQUAT

**Workouts A and B: 4x5-7**

*This exercise primarily works the quads, hamstrings, adductors, and glutes, but it also works the core (i.e., abs and lower back), from having to stabilize.*

- Hold a kettlebell or dumbbell against your chest, just below your chin. It will stay in this position at all times.
- Set your feet about shoulder-width apart or a bit wider, toes pointed out to the sides about ten to thirty degrees. Squat stance is very individual; play around and see what feels best—you may want your feet a bit wider, or a bit closer.
- To lock your back in a neutral, rigid position, push your chest out slightly and hold the bell against your chest. Maintain this rigid, neutral spine throughout the entire movement—no rounding the chest forward or hyperextending the lower back: keep the back rigid, like a crowbar.
- Begin the descent by sticking your butt back and bending the knees. As you squat down, keep your knees in line with your toes (knees shouldn't cave in toward each other). Control the lowering portion of the movement, keeping the back rigid. Lower until the crease in your

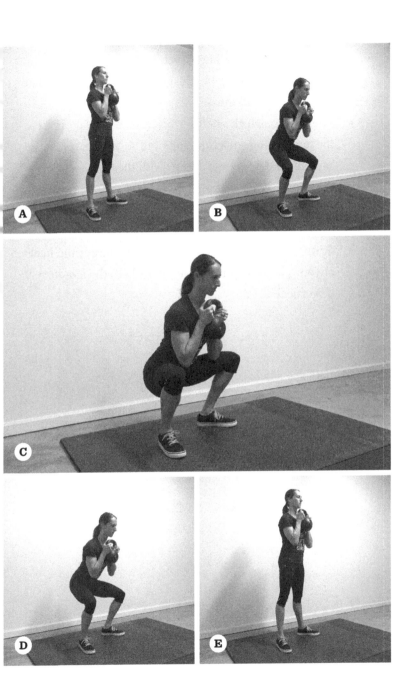

hips is a little below knee level, or the tops of the thighs are just below parallel to the ground. Feet should be flat on the floor at all times.

- After you reach the bottom position, smoothly reverse the motion and squat up—hips and shoulders rise at the same time, knees track in line with the toes, feet flat on the floor.
- Helpful cues: The kettlebell or dumbbell should travel in a vertical path between your feet when you lower down and squat up. If using a dumbbell, put the heels of your palms under one end of the bell; the handle will be vertical.

It's okay for the knees to go over your toes, as long as you apply the coaching cues. Everyone's squat will look a little different, depending on limb and torso length.

If using a dumbbell, put the heels of your palms under one of the ends. The handle will be vertical to the ground. If using a kettlebell (like in the photo) hold it by the "horns."

Think of your back as a crowbar. You want it locked in a neutral, rigid position. Don't allow it to hyperextend or flex during the movement.

## What to Watch Out For
The biggest mistakes in the goblet squat are flexing or extending the back, and letting the knees cave in. Those are the things

that cause pain. If your back stays locked in a neutral, rigid position and your knees track in line with your toes throughout the entire movement (on the way down and when squatting back up), you shouldn't feel discomfort.

## PUSH-UP

Workout A: 4x5-7

*This exercise primarily works the chest, anterior shoulders, and triceps. It also works the core from stabilizing the body.*

Regardless of whether you can perform push-ups on the ground or you perform the elevated version (with a barbell set securely in a power rack, demonstrated here, or with a Smith machine), the same cues apply. For sake of the example, I'll refer specifically to an elevated push-up. The elevated version is superior to push-ups performed on the knees because there's more core engagement, and it's best for progressing to traditional push-ups.

- The higher the bar, the easier the movement will be (you'll lift less of your bodyweight). Better to start with the bar too high—you can always lower it to make the movement more challenging.
- Grab the bar with hands a bit wider than shoulder-width apart, and keep the wrists mostly neutral (don't let them hyperextend). Your body should be in a straight line from the top of your head to your ankles, *and it should remain in this position at all times.* To help maintain this rigid position, squeeze your stomach and butt. Note: A slight bend in the knees is fine if having them fully extended causes discomfort.

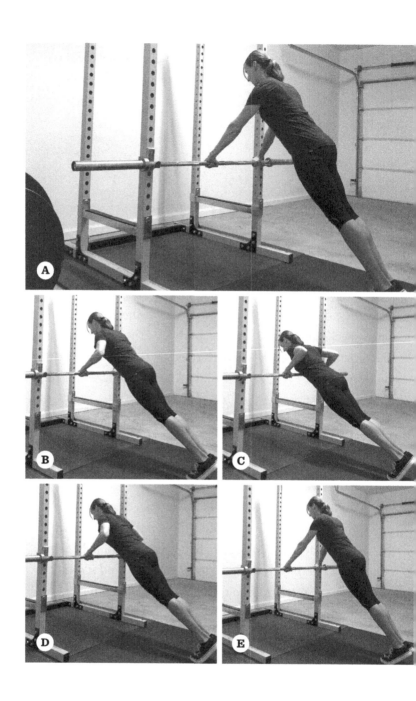

- Keeping your body straight, bend your elbows to lower yourself to the bar. Upper arms should be at an approximately seventy-five-degree angle to your torso as you lower down. If viewed from above, your body would be in the shape of an arrow, not a T.
- Once the mid-chest lightly touches the bar, press back up to the start position.
- Remember, the body should remain in a straight line from the top of your head to your ankles. If you find your hips dropping or your chest coming up before your hips as you press back up, you need to raise the bar to make the movement easier.
- Note: Make sure the bar is securely placed in a power rack so it can't hop out of the supports.

For elevated push-ups and inverted rows, use a barbell set securely in a power rack, or a Smith machine. Not sure what those are? Get the resource guide at *www.niashanks.com/book-resource-guide/*.

## What to Watch Out For

Common mistakes include letting the hips sag when pressing back up. If this happens, you need to elevate the bar to make the movement easier, so you can keep your body locked in a straight, neutral position. The other mistake is lowering the upper chest to the bar while your arms flare out to ninety degrees. Aiming the mid-chest to the bar will ensure the upper arms are closer to a seventy-five-degree angle to the torso, which is more shoulder-friendly.

For all exercises, keep your neck neutral (i.e., in line with your spine). Don't hyperextend your neck, and don't turn your head while performing an exercise. That's how you can strain a muscle.

## INVERTED ROW
**Workout A: 4x5-7**

*This exercise primarily works the back, posterior deltoids, biceps, and forearms. It also works the core from having to stabilize the body.*

It helps many trainees to think of this movement as a reverse push-up. Whereas with a push-up you push your body away from the bar, with the inverted row you pull your body *to* the bar.

- Use a barbell set securely in a power rack, or Smith machine; the higher the bar, the easier the movement will be. Better to start with the bar too high than too low.
- Grab the bar with hands a little wider than shoulder-width apart, and walk your feet forward. As with the push-up, your body should be in a straight line from the top of your head to your ankles (a slight bend in the knees is fine if having them extended causes discomfort). To maintain this straight, rigid position, squeeze your stomach and butt.

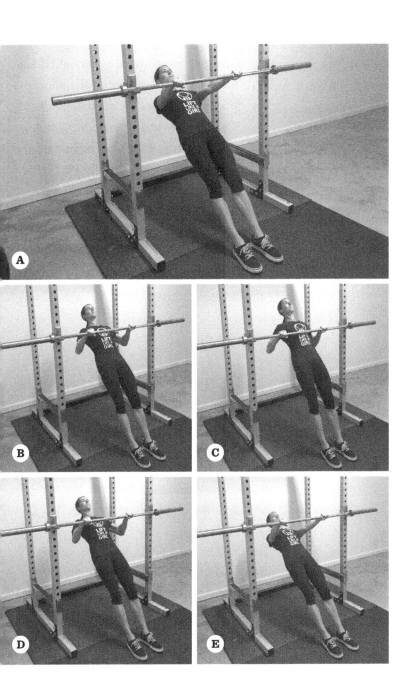

The feet may slide out of place. If that happens, put something there to help hold your feet in place.

- Keep your body in a straight line, and pull your body up to the bar; upper arms will be at approximately a seventy-five-degree angle to your torso. At the top of the movement the bar should hit the mid-chest; if it's higher than this, you need to walk your feet back a few inches.
- Once the mid-chest touches the bar, lower your body down under control, keeping your body in a straight line.
- If you can't keep your body in a straight line (your hips drop to the ground), you need to raise the height of the bar to make the movement easier.

Some people find when they pull their body up to the bar it touches their neck. If that happens, you're too far under the bar and need to walk back and try the movement again. The bar should touch the mid-chest.

How to improve performance with push-ups and inverted rows: Once you perform seven reps for all four sets, lower the bar a little to make the movement more challenging (you'll lift a greater percentage of your bodyweight). For example, if you had a barbell on number 12 of the power rack, lower it to 11 the following workout. Note: if the holes aren't numbered on the power rack or Smith machine, count up starting from the bottom hole and record this in your workout log.

# ROMANIAN DEADLIFT (RDL)

## Workout B: 4x5-7

*This exercise is what's known as a "hip hinge" movement, and it primarily works the glutes, hamstrings, and lower back (also referred to as the posterior chain). It also works the upper back and is great for building grip strength.*

- Set a barbell in a rack so it's about an inch or two above knee level. You will take the bar out of the rack to start this movement (so you begin from the top of the exercise).
- Grab the bar so your hands are shoulder-width apart on the bar (they should be close to perpendicular to the ground, just outside your thighs). Put your feet under the bar at hip-width, so the bar is above the mid-foot. To get the bar out of the rack, lock your back in a neutral position, stand up straight, and keep the bar over the mid-foot; take one small step back with one foot, and then with the other. This part is not shown in the photos.
- Set your feet about hip-width apart (feet are closer together than with a squat), toes pointed straight ahead. The bar should be against your thighs and directly over the mid-foot (i.e., the arches).
- The bar will travel over the mid-foot throughout the entire movement.
- Squeeze the bar hard, and push your chest out slightly to lock the back in a neutral, rigid position (you will maintain this rigid torso throughout the entire

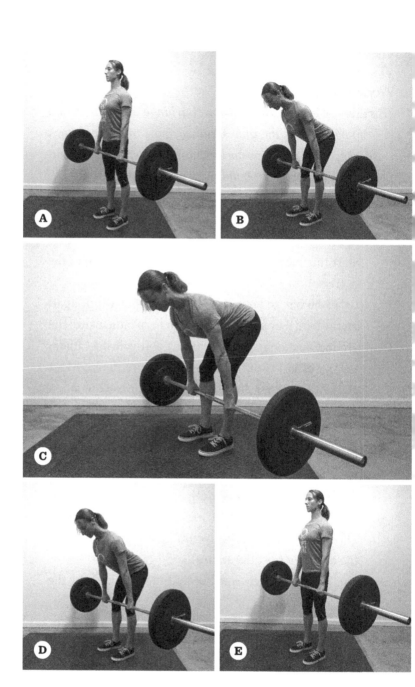

movement—your chest shouldn't round forward, and your lower back shouldn't hyperextend).

- Push the hips back to lower the bar; the knees will bend a bit more as the bar approaches and passes the kneecaps. Again, the bar should travel over the mid-foot. Lower the bar until it's a few inches below the kneecaps (about mid-shin or a little higher).

- Your torso should remain rigid at all times, like a crowbar. The movement should come from the hips—the position of the back shouldn't change (no flexing or extending).

- Once the bar is a few inches below the kneecaps, reverse the motion; keep the bar over the mid-foot, and push the hips forward to raise the bar.

- Return to a tall standing position; do not lean back.

- When all reps are completed, put the bar back in the rack.

- Do you have trouble holding on to the bar? As the weight gets heavier, your grip may give out. Use a double-overhand grip (used in photos) for all warm-up sets and for as many work sets as possible. If your grip is limiting the weight you can handle, use a mixed grip: one palm will face up, the other will face down. Switch your hands each set. You can also use straps; this is explained in the free resource guide (www.niashanks.com/book-resource-guide/).

For barbell exercises (RDL in Phase 1; squat, deadlift, standing press, and bench press in Phase 2), calculate the weight lifted by adding the weight of the barbell and the plates loaded on it. Most standard barbells weigh forty-five pounds. So if you performed RDLs with a standard barbell with a ten-pound plate on each side, you lifted sixty-five pounds.

### What to Watch Out For

A common mistake with the RDL is letting the bar drift over the toes. Make sure the bar travels over the mid-foot in a vertical line on the way down and on the way up.

Some people tend to lean back once they finish the movement. Don't lean back at the top—the rep is complete when you're standing straight up.

Some people look up to the ceiling during this exercise; this hyperextends the neck. Keep the neck in line with the back. Stare at a spot on the floor about ten to twenty feet in front of you.

## STANDING DUMBBELL PRESS

### Workout B: 4x5-10

*This exercise primarily works the shoulders and triceps, but it also works the abs, back, glutes, and legs from having to stabilize.*

Stand tall with feet about shoulder-width apart. Get your

entire body tight: Squeeze your stomach, quads, and glutes, and keep them squeezed the entire time. You want your entire body braced and rigid.

- With your body tight, begin with the dumbbells near chin level, hands in a neutral grip (palms facing each other), elbows slightly in front of the body (not flared out to the sides). Forearms should be perpendicular to the ground, and wrists mostly straight (not hyperextended).

- Press the dumbbells straight up over your head, and shrug your shoulders at the top of the movement to complete the lift, like you're trying to punch the ceiling. Lower under control, returning the dumbbells to about chin level. The bells should travel in a vertical line.

- Helpful cue: Keep your whole body braced the entire time, and actively squeeze your stomach, quads, and glutes.

The exception to the standard number of reps is the standing dumbbell press. Perform four sets of five to ten reps. Because most dumbbells increase in five-pound increments, it may be tough to do four sets of seven reps with a fifteen-pound dumbbell and next time move up to twenty; the increase could be too much. Stick with a weight until you do four sets of ten reps for the standing dumbbell press. The next workout, increase the weight and go back to five reps.

A helpful cue to maintain a rigid tightness is to act like someone is going to push you. You'd naturally brace for that. Staying tight provides a more stable

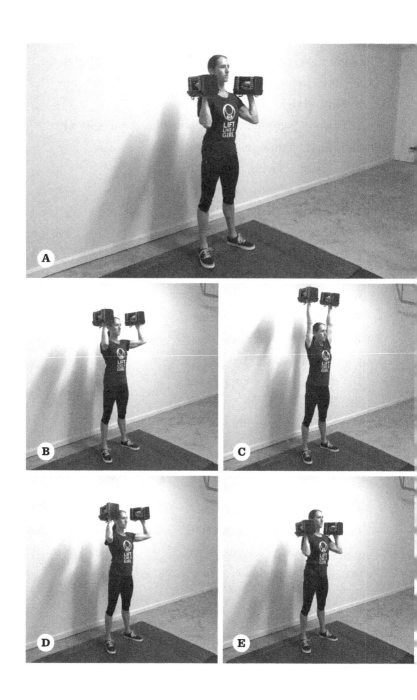

base for pressing a weight overhead. This becomes even more important when you use a barbell in Phase 2.

Shrugging the traps at the top of the movement helps prevent shoulder impingement. This is a great coaching cue from Mark Rippetoe in *Starting Strength Basic Barbell Training, Third Edition.*

## NOTES ON PHASE I

Now that you've seen Workouts A and B for Phase 1, and know how to correctly perform each exercise, here's some additional information for how to perform, and progress, the workouts.

- After completing the general warm-up and the warm-ups sets for the first exercise, perform the first exercise for four sets of five to seven reps, with the same weight on all sets. Then repeat the process with the remaining exercises.

- For Workout A, perform all four sets of goblet squats on its own, then move on to push-ups and inverted rows. You can perform push-ups and inverted rows as a superset, performing them in alternating fashion. Perform a set of push-ups, rest as needed, perform a set of inverted rows, rest as needed, and repeat until you perform four sets for both exercises. You don't have to do them as a superset, but it's more efficient.

- For Workout B, perform all sets for each exercise on their own. That means you'll perform four sets for RDLs (this does not include warm-up sets), then four sets of standing dumbbell presses, and finish with four sets of goblet squats.

- You must improve your performance! The workouts use the double-progression method to accomplish this mandatory goal. Start at the low end of the provided rep range—five reps. Use the same weight for all work sets, and stick with that weight until you perform the high end of the provided rep range for all sets—seven (except for the standing dumbbell press, which is ten).

Then, once you perform the high end of the provided rep range with the same weight for all sets, increase the weight about five pounds the following workout (you may be able to add ten pounds to the RDL the first couple of workouts), and start back at the low end of the provided rep range—five. Remember, improve your performance with push-ups and inverted rows by gradually lowering the bar, thus lifting a greater percentage of your bodyweight. Keep repeating in this fashion. That's what makes this a double-progression. You start out performing more reps with the same weight, and then increase the weight. Some exercises will progress quicker than others, which is perfectly fine.

Reminder: If you're new to strength training, or you're coming back after a layoff, begin by performing two sets for each exercise instead of four. Do this the first week, and if you don't get too sore, perform three sets the following week. By the third week of training, you should be able to perform four sets for all exercises. It's better to start out conservative, because you can always progress the following workout.

- Rest periods between sets of an exercise will vary, but you'll likely only need to rest about forty-five to sixty seconds between sets for the first couple of weeks. Once you get stronger and use heavier weights, you may need closer to ninety seconds. Rule of thumb: Rest as long as needed to put full effort into the next set.

- Stick with Phase 1 for at least four weeks (if you're not new to strength training) or upwards of eight to twelve weeks (if you are new to strength training or when you struggle to progress on most exercises). Then move on to Phase 2.

- Keep a workout log! Record your workouts so you know exactly what weight you used and how many reps you performed (do not rely on memory). This way, you know exactly what needs to be done to beat your performance when you repeat the workout. It's also helpful to keep notes in the workout log (e.g., *Everything felt strong today; I really needed to focus on making sure my knees tracked in line with my toes on squats; I set a personal record*, etc.). Get a cheap composite notebook, or use your favorite app. Just be sure to track everything. The workout log is fun, and motivating, to flip through after you've been training for several months; you'll see how much stronger you've become. Bottom line: It doesn't matter how you record your workouts, just make sure you do.

## QUALITY IS SUPERIOR TO QUANTITY

*Lift Like a Girl* is built around using high-efficiency exercises, the fewest movements that will deliver the best results, instead of performing dozens of exercises. So yes, you're only doing three exercises per workout. Fewer exercises means you'll be able to maintain focus for the entire workout, and you'll learn proper technique quicker, and get stronger faster, because you're doing the same movements frequently.

### LIFT LIKE A GIRL IN REAL LIFE

"In a very short time span of three months, I'm seeing noticeable muscle definition along with an increase in strength. My form on all exercises is getting better, along with my posture. My knees, back, shoulders (which I've always had some discomfort with) feel healthy and virtually pain-free! For the first time in five years, I'm learning that *quality* trumps quantity. One of the best aspects of Nia's program is the simplicity of it. I will admit that at first I was a little skeptical that only a few basic movements would provide such impressive results. I learned very quickly that to perform these movements with excellent form is not only super effective, but *hard* and challenging. To sum it up, I'm in love with this program and I'm *so* happy to have found Nia. I get excited when I know I get to train! Adding weight to the bar, getting stronger, performing more push-ups and chin-ups, all those goals are incredibly satisfying and make training *fun*. My ultimate goal is not to look a particular way or compare myself to anyone; it is to become the strongest version of *me*."

Exercise variety and rarely repeating the same workout is part of a current fitness craze. Some people claim muscle confusion is necessary for achieving the best results (it's not) and that's why they rotate exercises frequently. There's one huge problem with this approach, beyond the myth it perpetuates: If you constantly change exercises, you can't accurately track progress. How will you know if you're getting stronger if you constantly change your workouts? There are too many variables to track.

You may think you'll get mind-numbingly bored from repeating the same two workouts in Phases 1 and 2. Remember, the ultimate goal of the strength training programs is to build strength, hone proper technique, and deliver the best possible results with the fewest exercises and workouts necessary. In order to achieve that goal, you need to use big compound movements, train them frequently, and steadily improve performance. There's nothing boring about getting stronger and discovering what your body is capable of doing, especially as you get closer to—and shatter—training milestones (e.g., busting out traditional push-ups, squatting the equivalent of your bodyweight, etc.). This also builds motivation to keep training, to get stronger, to become *more*.

## PHASE 1 TRAINING LOG EXAMPLE

Below is a sample training log that includes the elements discussed above: general warm-up, warm-up sets, rest periods between sets, cool-down, and how to improve your performance each time you repeat a workout over a two-week period.

**WEEK 1**

Workout A, Monday:

General warm-up: Walked on a treadmill for five minutes.

1. Goblet squat
- Warm-up set #1: 10 × 10 (10 pounds, 10 reps)
- Warm-up set #2: 20 × 5 (20 pounds, 5 reps)
  - Work set #1: 30 × 5, rest 60 seconds (30 pounds, 5 reps, rest 60 seconds)
  - Work set #2: 30 × 5, rest 60 seconds
  - Work set #3: 30 × 5, rest 60 seconds
  - Work set #4: 30 × 5, rest 60 seconds

2. Push-ups and inverted rows (exercises performed as a superset)
- Push-up warm-up set #1: 14 × 8 (barbell set in rack on 14th hole, 8 reps)
- Inverted row warm-up set #1: 15 × 8 (barbell set in rack on 15th hole, 8 reps)
  - Push-up work set #1: 9 × 5, rest 45 seconds (barbell set in rack on 9th hole, 5 reps)
  - Inverted row work set #1: 10 × 5, rest 45 seconds (barbell set in rack on 10th hold, 5 reps)
  - Push-up work set #2: 9 × 5, rest 45 seconds
  - Inverted row work set #2: 10 × 5, rest 45 seconds
  - Push-up work set #3: 9 × 5, rest 45 seconds
  - Inverted row work set #3: 10 × 5, rest 45 seconds
  - Push-up work set #4: 9 × 5, rest 45 seconds
  - Inverted row work set #4: 10 × 5, rest 45 seconds

Cool-down: Walked around the gym for five minutes.

Workout B, Wednesday:

General warm-up: Walked on a treadmill for five minutes.

1. RDL
- Warm-up set #1: 45 × 10 (45 pounds, 10 reps)
- Warm-up set #2: 65 × 5 (65 pounds, 5 reps)
    - Work set #1: 85 × 5, rest 75 seconds (85 pounds, 5 reps, rest 75 seconds)
    - Work set #2: 85 × 5, rest 75 seconds
    - Work set #3: 85 × 5, rest 75 seconds
    - Work set #4: 85 × 5, rest 75 seconds

2. Standing dumbbell press
- Warm-up set #1: 5 × 8 (5 pounds, 8 reps)
    - Work set #1: 10 × 5, rest 60 seconds (10 pounds, 5 reps, rest 60 seconds)
    - Work set #2: 10 × 5, rest 60 seconds
    - Work set #3: 10 × 5, rest 60 seconds
    - Work set #4: 10 × 5, rest 60 seconds

3. Goblet squat
- Warm-up set #1: 10 × 10 (10 pounds, 10 reps)
- Warm-up set #2: 20 × 5 (20 pounds, 5 reps)
    - Work set #1: 30 × 7, rest 60 seconds
    - Work set #2: 30 × 7, rest 60 seconds
    - Work set #3: 30 × 7, rest 60 seconds
    - Work set #4: 30 × 7, rest 60 seconds

Cool-down: Walked around the gym for five minutes.

It's important to note that the goblet squat is performed in both workouts, so you'll improve your performance with this exercise every workout. The same weight was used from Monday's workout, but two more reps were performed for each set, reaching the high end of the provided rep range (seven, for this exercise). The weight will be increased for goblet squats on Friday's workout.

## Workout A, Friday

General warm-up, warm-up sets, and cool-down are not shown for brevity, but should still be performed:

1. Goblet squat: 35 x 4 x 5, 60 seconds rest (35 pounds, 4 sets, 5 reps per set, rest 60 seconds between sets)
2. Push-up: 9 x 4 x 7, 45 seconds rest (barbell was set in rack on 9th hole, 4 sets, 7 reps per set, rest 45 seconds between sets)
3. Inverted row: 10 x 4 x 7, 45 seconds rest (barbell was set in rack on 10th hold, 4 sets, 7 reps per set, rest 45 seconds between sets)

Our trainee improved her performance on all exercises: She added five pounds to the goblet squats from the previous workout and returned to the low end of the provided rep range. She reached the high end of the provided rep range for push-ups and inverted rows. Next workout she'll lower the barbell in the rack to make the push-ups and inverted rows more challenging, and return to the low end of the rep range—five.

You don't have to rest exactly sixty or forty-five seconds between sets. This is just an example. The first couple of weeks you may only need forty-five to sixty seconds of rest between sets, but as you get stronger and the weights get heavier, you may want closer to seventy-five to ninety seconds of rest.

## WEEK 2

Workout B, Monday

General warm-up, warm-up sets, and cool-down are not shown, but should still be performed:

1. RDL: 85 x 4 x 7, 75 seconds rest (85 pounds, 4 sets, 7 reps per set, 75 seconds rest between sets)
2. Standing dumbbell press: 10 x 4 x 8, 60 seconds rest (10 pounds, 4 sets, 8 reps per set, 60 seconds rest between sets)
3. Goblet squat: 35 x 4 x 6, 60 seconds rest (35 pounds, 4 sets, 6 reps per set, 60 seconds rest between sets)

The high end of the rep range was reached for RDLs, so the trainee will increase the weight the following workout and go back to five reps per set. For the dumbbell press, she'll stick with the same weight the following workout, until she completes ten reps per set for this exercise; then she'll add weight and go back to five reps. She improved her performance for the goblet squats by performing one more rep per set than last time. Since she got six reps per set, she'll stick with the same weight for the next workout.

> There's no hard-set rule on how many reps to add each workout. If you started with five reps the first workout, and you know you can perform seven reps when you repeat it, then do seven instead of just six. Likewise, if you know the weight was very light when you reach the high end of the rep range, you can increase the weight ten pounds instead of five for the following workout.

## Workout A, Wednesday

General warm-up, warm-up sets, and cool-down are not shown, but should still be performed:

1. Goblet squat: 35 x 4 x 7, 60 seconds rest (35 pounds, 4 sets, 7 reps per set, rest 60 seconds between sets)
2. Push-up: 8 x 4 x 5, 45 seconds rest (barbell was lowered to 8th hole in power rack, 4 sets, 5 reps per set, rest 45 seconds between sets)
3. Inverted row: 9 x 4 x 5, 45 seconds rest (barbell was lowered to 9th hole in power rack, 4 sets, 5 reps per set, rest 45 seconds between sets)

The trainee reached the high end of the rep range for goblet squats, so the weight will be increased the next workout.

The bar was lowered for push-ups and inverted rows, so she returned to the low end of the rep range; this same bar height will be used the following workout, and more reps per set will be performed.

## Workout B, Friday

General warm-up, warm-up sets, and cool-down are not shown, but should still be performed:

> 1. RDL: 90 x 4 x 5, 75 seconds rest (90 pounds, 4 sets, 5 reps per set, 75 seconds rest between sets)
> 2. Dumbbell press: 10 x 4 x 10, 60 seconds rest (10 pounds, 4 sets, 10 reps per set, 60 seconds rest between sets)
> 3. Goblet squat: 40 x 4 x 5, 60 seconds rest (40 pounds, 4 sets, 5 reps per set, 60 seconds rest between sets)

Weight was added to RDLs, so the trainee returned to the low end of the rep range, five reps per set. She reached the high end of the rep range for the dumbbell press (ten for this exercise), so she'll increase the weight the next workout. Weight was added to goblet squats, so the trainee returned to the low end of the provided rep range.

A trainee who is brand new to strength training will continue following Phase 1 in this fashion for approximately eight to twelve weeks (or whenever they can no longer make progress on most exercises) and then move on to Phase 2. Someone who is not new to strength training can move on to Phase 2 after following Phase 1 for four weeks.

# LIFT LIKE A GIRL PHASE 2

Once you've followed Phase 1 for four to twelve weeks (depending on your experience level when you started), it's time to move on to Phase 2.

Phase 2 transitions to exercises that allow for a greater loading potential—this means more barbell exercises, which are more scalable and allow for consistent loading. You can add more weight to a barbell squat than a goblet squat, for example. You'll be using exercise variations that allow for the most weight to be used. Deadlifts can handle the most weight followed by squats, bench presses, and then standing presses.

Perform three workouts per week, alternating Workout A and Workout B on nonconsecutive days, just like you did for Phase 1.

Phase 2 is very similar in fashion to Phase 1—you'll just be using different exercises. Every exercise has a rep range: Begin at the low end of the rep range and use the same weight for all work sets. Remember, warm-up sets are not shown in the workouts, but you need to do them. Once you complete the high end of the rep range with the same weight for all sets, add about five pounds (you may be able to add ten pounds the first few times to squats and deadlifts) to the next workout, and start back at the low end of the rep range. Continue repeating this sequence.

Practice the same habits you built with Phase 1. Begin each workout with a general warm-up, and warm-up for each exercise as you did in Phase 1. Remember, exercises that allow for more weight to be used may require an extra warm-up set or two, and as you progress through Phase 2 and get stronger, you may want to add an extra warm-up set.

Perform all sets of an exercise on its own before moving on to the next one in the workout. Finally, conclude each workout with a brief cool-down for about five minutes.

### *LIFT LIKE A GIRL* PHASE 2 WORKOUTS
Workout A:
1. Squat: 4x5-7
2. Bench press: 4x5-7
3. Chin-up/pull-down: 4x5-7

Bench Press Workout Tip

If you're not comfortable performing the bench press or you'd rather reach the milestone of performing a flawless set of traditional push-ups, stick with push-ups from Phase 1 and pick up where you left off with them. However, once you perform 4x7 of traditional push-ups, it's recommended you move on to the bench press. It's easier to progressively load the barbell bench press; loading a push-up can be difficult and awkward.

Chin-Up Workout Tip

Most trainees will not be able to perform chin-ups from the beginning. Not a problem! If possible, perform assisted chin-ups: loop a resistance band through itself around the chin-up bar, and put your feet in the band. If this is too challenging at first, or you don't have the equipment, substitute cable pull-downs. Most gyms have a cable machine you sit in, with a pad resting on the top of your thighs. If you choose to use the cable machine, use the shoulder-width, palms-up grip. If you start with cable pull-downs, aim to get as strong as you can with them, and then switch to assisted chin-ups when possible.

Workout B:

    I. Deadlift/RDL*: 4x5-6

    2. Standing barbell press: 4x5-7

    3. One-arm dumbbell row: 4x7-12

\*     After performing Phase 2 for at least eight weeks, you have the option to alternate deadlifts and RDLs each time you repeat Workout B. If after a couple of months on Phase 2 you feel like deadlifting that frequently is too challenging to recover from (because the deadlift allows for a lot of weight to be used), you can alternate RDLs with the deadlifts. For example, if you do Workout B on Monday and again on Friday, deadlift Monday and perform RDLs on Friday, and then deadlift again on Wednesday. Keep alternating in this fashion.

## SQUAT

Workout A: 4x5-7

*This exercise primarily works the quads, adductors, hamstrings, and glutes, but it also works the lower back and abs.*

This replaces the goblet squat from Phase 1. One big change you'll notice (other than having a barbell on your back) is that, unlike the goblet squat, your torso will *not* maintain such a vertical angle. Due to the bar placement, you will lean forward a bit more as you squat down. Some people think this means they're doing the movement wrong because they're

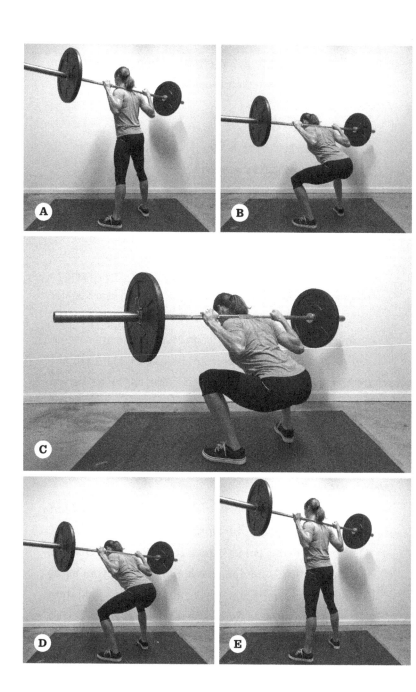

used to being more upright with the goblet squat, but it's just part of the exercise.

- Use proper safety measures. Perform squats in a power rack with safety bars: Set them a couple of inches below where the barbell will be when you're at the bottom of the squat. This way, just in case something goes wrong, the safety bars will catch the barbell. Many people squat outside of a rack and "dump" the bar if something goes wrong. I'm not going to tell you how to do this, because I recommend using a rack and safety bars to instill confidence.

  It's okay for the knees to go over the toes; this is not a problem. Everyone's squat will look a little different because of individual limb and torso length. Just be sure to follow the provided coaching cues.

- Set the bar in a rack so it's about upper chest level. (You want to be able to get the bar out of the rack easily—you shouldn't have to get on your tiptoes to get it out of the rack.) Take the closest grip you comfortably can—a little wider than shoulder-width—and get under the bar; pinch your shoulder blades together (which helps maintain a tight upper back). The bar should be on your traps *below your C7 vertebrae* (the bony prominence at the base of your neck—you do not want the bar resting on this).
- Have your feet under your shoulders; the bar should be in line with the mid-foot. Squat the bar up out of the

supports. Take a step back with one leg, and then bring the other back. Be efficient—you want to take the fewest steps necessary. This becomes more important as the weight gets heavier.

- Set your feet. A good starting point is feet shoulder-width apart, give or take a bit, toes pointed out to the sides about ten to thirty degrees. The setup will be similar to what you used for the goblet squat, but you may want to play with your stance a little to find what's comfortable.

*If the palms-up grip causes wrist or elbow pain/discomfort, use a neutral grip—palms facing each other.*

- With feet set, it's time to get your entire body tight. Push your chest out slightly (shoulder blades should still be pulled together), take a breath, and brace your abs (imagine someone is about to punch you in the stomach)—to get a neutral, rigid back. As you squat down, you want to maintain a neutral spine: You don't want the upper back rounding forward, nor the lower back extending. Tight, rigid, neutral spine is what you want throughout the entire movement.

- Pick a spot to stare at. Some people prefer looking straight ahead, while others like to look at a spot on the floor about ten to twenty feet in front of them. Pick a spot, and focus on it.

- Initiate the squat by sticking your butt back and breaking at the knees.

- Control the lowering portion; keep the back rigid (like a

crowbar) and your entire body tight. Knees should track in line with the toes (don't let them cave in), and feet should be flat on the floor—knees may go over the toes, and this is perfectly fine.

- Squat down until the crease in your hips is a little lower than your knees or until the tops of your thighs are slightly below parallel to the ground.

- Once you hit this depth, smoothly reverse the motion and squat back up. Hips and shoulders should rise at the same time, and knees track in line with the toes, while feet remain flat on the floor.

What about shoes? A good start is a pair of flat-soled, non-compressible shoes. These are great for all exercises. Some people prefer weightlifting shoes with a raised heel for squats. More on this in the free resource guide (*www.niashanks.com/book-resource-guide/*).

- Once in the top starting position, reset before performing the next rep. Make sure your chest is pushed out a bit to lock the back in a neutral, rigid position. Bring your shoulder blades together; take a breath, brace your stomach, and squat down again for the next rep.

- Helpful tip: The bar should travel in a vertical path over the mid-foot at all times. Some people find it more comfortable to use a thumbless grip (thumbs wrapped around the bar on the same side as fingers)—this is personal preference, so do what feels best to you.

## What to Watch Out For

There are three common squat mistakes. One is allowing the knees to cave in toward each other. Make sure the knees track in line with the feet/toes at all times, on the way down and up. The second is allowing the hips to shoot up before the shoulders when coming back up. Make sure the shoulders and hips rise out of the bottom at the same time. The third is allowing the bar to get out over the toes. The bar should travel in a vertical path over the mid-foot. To make sure you're doing this correctly, have someone watch you, or record your sets to see for yourself.

Think of your entire torso as a crowbar. As you squat down, keep your spine locked in a neutral, rigid position. You don't want the upper back rounding, or lower back extending. You want a rigid spine. Notice in the photos that the torso does lean forward during the descent, but there's no movement in the spine: It's locked in a neutral, rigid position on the way down and up.

A helpful cue when squatting back up is to think of driving your traps into the bar, and pushing the floor away from you. This is a cue courtesy of coach Tony Gentilcore.

Pause at the top before each rep. Lower down, squat up, and make sure your body is tight, and your back is locked in a neutral, rigid position—reset if you have to. Push your chest out slightly, pull the shoulder blades together, and brace your stomach. Then squat down again.

# BENCH PRESS

## Workout A: 4x5-7

*This exercise primarily works the chest, triceps, and anterior deltoids (i.e., front of the shoulders).*

This replaces the push-up from Phase 1. Before we go over how to perform this lift, ensure that you use proper safety measures:

- Have a competent spotter or, if you train alone, perform this exercise in a power rack with safety bars. Set the safety bars so they'll be about one inch lower than the bar when it's at the bottom position of the bench press. Because your back will be arched, you should be able to flatten out and have the bar rest on the safety bars. If you train alone, don't put collars on the sleeves of the barbell. This way, if necessary, you could dump the plates.
- Keep your feet flat on the floor, always.
- Wrap your thumb *around the bar* (i.e., opposite side of fingers). Do *not* do a thumbless grip on the bench press—this is unsafe.
- When you take the bar out of the rack, do so with focus.
- When you finish the set and are ready to rerack the bar, *lock it out above your shoulders first*. Finish the last rep and *then*, once your arms are locked out, guide it back into the safety hooks. Too many people start pushing the bar back toward the safety hooks on the last rep. Don't do this. Lock it out first and then take it back.

Here's how to perform the bench press:

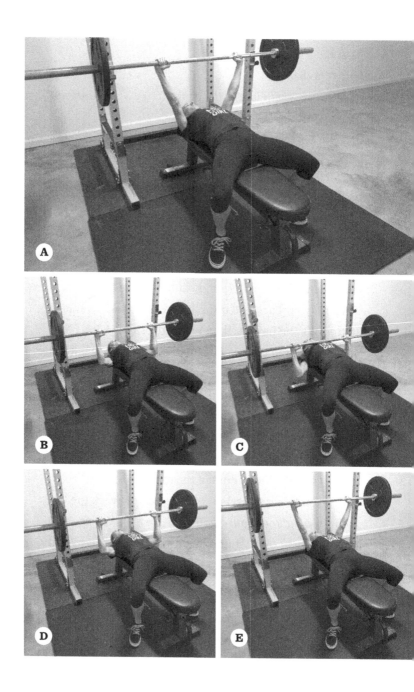

- Set up so your eyes are under the bar or a little below it, toward your feet. Feet should be planted firmly on the ground—some people prefer to have their shins perpendicular to the floor; others prefer to have them pulled back a few inches toward the head. Grab the bar a little wider than shoulder-width apart, about an inch or two wider on each side.

- Squeeze your shoulder blades together—act like you're trying to pinch a pencil between them. Keep them in this position throughout the set—don't let them come apart when bench pressing. This gives you a stable base to press from. Note: Make sure the bar isn't too high in the rack so you lose this upper-back tightness when you take the bar out of the rack. As you do this, stick your chest up toward the ceiling to get a small arch in your back.

Not confident to perform the bench press just yet? Stick with push-ups from Phase I until you can do 4x7 with your hands on the ground (i.e., traditional push-ups). Then switch to the bench press.

- With your feet planted firmly on the ground, shoulder blades pulled together, an arch in your lower back, and eyes under the barbell or a bit lower, press the barbell up out of the safety hooks and guide it, under control, over your shoulders. Wrists shouldn't be hyperextended—they'll have a bit of extension, but shouldn't be folded back. The barbell should be in line with the forearms.

- Lower the bar, under control, to the mid-chest—the

upper arms should be at about a seventy-five-degree angle to your torso (just like with push-ups in Phase 1—the bottom position of the bench press, viewed from above, should form an arrow shape, not a T, which can be hard on the shoulders).

- Once the bar lightly touches the mid-chest, press back up.
- Once you complete the final rep and the bar is locked out above your shoulders, guide the bar back into the safety hooks.

You may have seen powerlifters bench press with a ginormous arch in their back. Don't do that; we're not powerlifting. You want a small arch; you should easily be able to slide your hand under your lower back. The other benefit of the arch is that, should you use safety bars in a power rack set to the point if you flattened out your back, the barbell would rest on the safety pins.

# CHIN-UP/PULL-DOWN

## Workout A: 4x5-7

*This exercise primarily works the back, biceps, posterior deltoids, and forearms.*

If you can't (yet!) perform bodyweight chin-ups, use resistance bands for assistance (loop it through itself around the chin-up bar). Some gyms have assisted pull-up machines; that's fine too. Use a full range of motion, and make your muscles do the work. Don't just "fall" into the bottom position; lower yourself under complete control. If you have a good amount of weight to lose or don't have access to resistance bands, perform the cable pull-down (this is also a good exercise to start with to build confidence). If you choose to start with the cable pull-down, get as strong as you can with that exercise, and then progress to assisted chin-ups.

- Grab the bar with a shoulder-width, palms-up grip.
- If doing a chin-up, pull yourself up to the bar until your chin clears it, then slowly lower under control. To build strength with this movement, take a solid three seconds to lower down.
- Go all the way down. Half reps don't count.
- Thicker bands provide more assistance. Start with the thickest band you need until you complete four sets of seven reps, and then move to a smaller band and start back at five reps. Keep repeating until you're using the smallest available band.
- The goal of band-assisted chin-ups is to progress to not needing them. Once you're successfully using a very

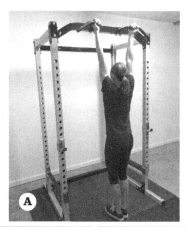

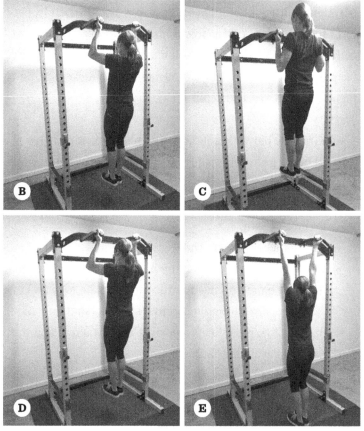

small band, start doing negatives; lower yourself down, from the top of the chin-up, under your own control with no assistance. Progress to being able to lower yourself taking a solid five seconds for every rep. Once you can do this for several reps, you'll be extremely close to being able to do an unassisted chin-up. To get back to the top after performing a negative, hop back up. It helps to have a sturdy box beneath your feet to make getting back to the top easier. Another option is to perform these in a Smith machine or with a barbell set securely in a power rack so it's about even with the top of your head. This way, you can perform the negative portion and then easily start back at the top.

Get the free resource guide for information on how to use resistance bands for assisted chin-ups at *www.niashanks.com/book-resource-guide/*.

- If you use a cable pull-down machine (not pictured), use the same grip described above, and pull the bar down until it just touches your clavicles. Resist the weight back up until your arms are completely straight.
- Note: If this grip causes wrist or elbow discomfort, switch to a neutral grip (palms facing each other). Keep your neck in a neutral position. Don't hyperextend your neck to get your chin over the bar. This is cheating and a good way to strain a muscle.

The palms-up grip is what makes this exercise a chin-up. A pull-up uses a palms-down grip. A neutral grip has palms facing each other.

If you're using resistance bands, make sure you control the lowering portion—take a solid three seconds to lower down. And don't stop halfway—you must go all the way back down for every rep.

## DEADLIFT

**Workout B: 4x5-6**

*This exercise primarily works the glutes, hamstrings, lower back, upper back, and forearms.*

- The correct stance will be what you used for the RDL in Phase 1: usually hip-width or a little narrower. Don't go too wide—this is a common mistake.
- Put your feet (using the stance determined above) under the bar until your shins are about one inch away from the bar. The bar should be over the arches of the feet—the mid-foot.
- Reach down and grab the bar—hands should be just outside the legs. You want the closest grip possible without your arms rubbing against your legs.
- Push your shins forward gently until they lightly touch the bar to drop the hips down, and then push your chest out to set the back in a rigid, neutral position.
- With the chest pushed out and back set in a neutral position, the hips will be lower than the shoulders and higher than the knees. Your back should be neutral and your

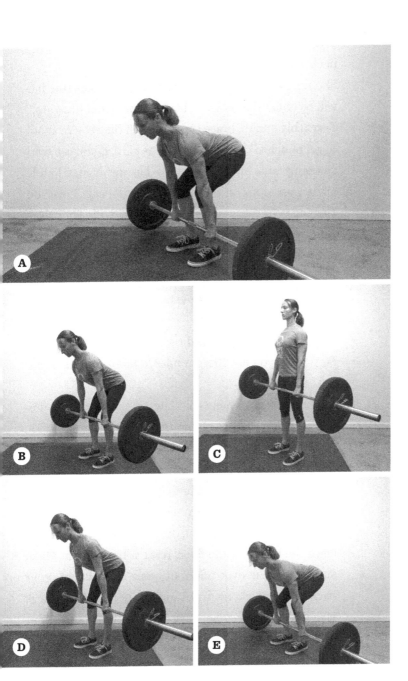

neck in line with the spine.

- Shoulders should be a little in front of the bar (the bar will be under the shoulder blades), and arms straight.

- Take a big breath, brace your stomach (like you're about to get punched), squeeze the bar as hard as you can, and smoothly pull (do *not* jerk) the bar up; it may lightly graze your shins on the way up. Helpful cue: Focus on keeping your chest pushed out, and drive the floor away from you.

- As the bar comes off the ground, it should travel over the mid-foot at all times, and the back should remain tight and rigid. No rounding or extending—think of it, again, like a crowbar.

- Hips and shoulders should rise at the same time.

- Stop when you are straight up—do *not* lean back at the top.

- Reverse the movement—initiate the lowering by sticking your butt back, keeping the bar over the mid-foot. Once the bar reaches about kneecap level, your knees will bend to lower the bar down.

- At the risk of sounding redundant: Keep the bar over the mid-foot. Keep your body tight and chest pushed out when lowering the bar back down under control.

- Once the bar is on the floor, reset your position. Make sure the bar is over mid-foot, your chest is out, your back is locked in a neutral, rigid position, and your neck is in line with the spine. Take a breath, brace your stomach, and repeat.

- Note: This is called a *dead*lift for a reason. Bring the bar to a complete rest on the ground before every rep. Do not bounce the bar off the floor between reps.

- Remember, the bar should travel in a vertical path over the mid-foot.
- Tip: Some trainees find it's more comfortable to point their toes out slightly at about a five- to fifteen-degree angle. It's a personal preference; you can try it with your toes straight ahead and pointed out to the sides slightly to see what you prefer.
- Friendly tip: The bar may be grazing your shins; wear pants or high socks when deadlifting.
- Grip tip: Use a double-overhand grip as long as possible. Most women (especially those with petite hands) will find they can't hold the bar this way as the weights get heavier. Use the double-overhand grip for as many warm-up and work sets as possible. Switch to the mixed grip (one palm up, the other palm down) when needed, and alternate the grip each set.

Having trouble getting your back locked into a rigid, neutral position? Elevate the plates one to four inches by stacking them on blocks, mats, or bumper plates. For someone who can't pull a barbell off the floor without losing tightness in their back, this solves the issue. Elevate to the lowest height possible. This means if you can get, and keep, your back locked in a neutral position by elevating the plates only two inches, don't elevate them four.

## What to Watch Out For

A common mistake is trying to squat the weight up, so people will drop their hips too low, like in the bottom of the squat. A helpful cue to prevent this: The barbell should be beneath your shoulder blades when you're setting up to perform a deadlift.

> If your gym doesn't have bumper plates (which are the same diameter regardless of weight), and you can't yet use a forty-five-pound plate on each side, you may need to elevate the plates so they reach the standard height; from the floor to the bottom of the barbell should be about eight and a half inches. Smaller iron plates increase the range of motion—this isn't a bad thing, but some people are unable to keep their back locked in a neutral, rigid position with an increased range of motion.

## What to Watch Out For

A common mistake is trying to jerk the bar off the ground. Keep your arms straight, and smoothly break the bar off the ground—don't jerk it. Another mistake is not keeping the back locked in a rigid, neutral position. When you set up, push your chest out to get your back in a neutral position; brace your stomach to help lock this position in place. The third mistake is allowing the hips to shoot up before the shoulders. When you pull the bar off the floor, hips and shoulders should rise at the same time.

# STANDING BARBELL PRESS

## Workout B: 4x5-7

*This exercise primarily works the shoulders and triceps, but the core (abs and lower back), glutes, and legs are involved to stabilize the body.*

This exercise replaces the standing dumbbell press performed in Phase 1.

- Set the bar in a power rack at the same height used for squats.
- Grab the bar so your hands are a little wider than shoulder-width apart (this will be a closer grip than used for the bench press). Get under the bar so it's over the mid-foot, squat up to get the bar out of the rack, and take one small step back with one foot, and then the other—be efficient.
- Elbows should be in front of your body (not out to the sides) and forearms perpendicular to the floor. Wrists will be extended slightly; don't let them fold back and hyperextend. The barbell should be in line with the forearms.
- Stand tall with feet about shoulder-width apart (most people find their squat stance a good place to set their feet). The bar should be a little over your shoulders or a little under your chin (this varies according to individual limb length).
- It's imperative to create total body tension. Squeeze your stomach, quads, and glutes, and keep them tight the entire time.

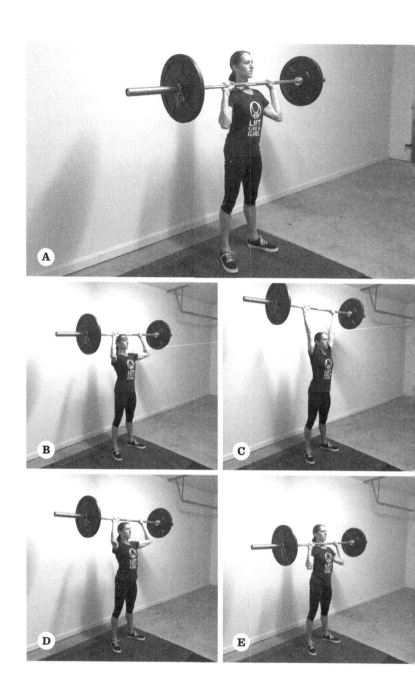

- From this position—stomach, glutes, and legs tight, elbows in front of the body—take a big breath and brace like you're about to get punched, then press the bar straight up. You'll have to pull your head back a bit so the bar doesn't hit your chin—this hurts, so don't do it.
- Bring your head back under the bar as it clears your head. At the top of the movement, shrug your shoulders up, like you're trying to punch the ceiling.
- Lower the bar under control, and get your head out of the way again.
- Helpful cue: Make sure your entire body is tight, with elbows in front of the body, take a big breath and brace your stomach, and then press. The bar will travel in a vertical path over the mid-foot at all times.

Fractional plates are going to be extremely useful for the barbell press. Out of all the barbell exercises used in Phase 2, this is the exercise that will have the slowest, and smallest, weight progression. You'll likely need to use one-pound weight increases after a couple of months of training, and then even half-pound increases.

After building pressing strength in Phase 1 with the dumbbell press, you've hopefully built enough strength to do this movement with a standard barbell at the gym. Standard barbells are forty-five pounds. For a very petite woman, though, this is probably going to be too much. In that case, she's going to have to use whatever smaller bar her gym has, until she can work up to the Olympic bar.

Wondering if you can use the Smith machine for the squat, deadlift, bench press, and standing press? If that's the only option, then yes. However, the Smith machine removes the stability, balance, and coordination components that are present with the barbell variations, since the barbell in the Smith machine moves in a fixed path on rails. For efficiency and effectiveness, the barbell variations are preferred.

## ONE-ARM DUMBBELL ROW
### Workout B: 4x7-12
*This exercise primarily works the back, biceps, posterior deltoids, and forearms (grip strength).*

- Put your knee and same-side hand on a bench. The other foot will be planted on the floor, and the other hand will be holding the dumbbell. Your torso will be almost parallel with the floor.
- Squeeze the dumbbell hard, and pull it up *toward your hip*. Lower under control until the arm is fully extended.
- Do all the reps for one side, and then do the same number of reps on the other. Start with the weaker arm.
- Helpful cue: Think about pulling your elbow up toward your hip. Keep your torso tight and rigid. A little movement is fine, but you shouldn't be twisting or jerking the weight.

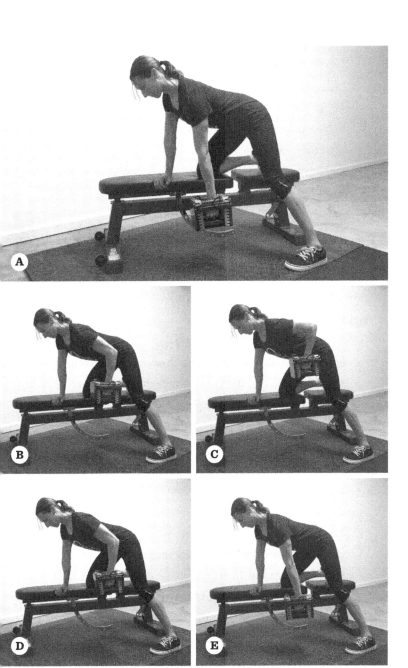

This exercise uses a wider rep range because most dumbbells increase in five-pound increments. Sticking with the same weight for a higher rep range makes those jumps more manageable. If you struggle to use a heavier dumbbell, stick with the same weight and continue adding reps until you no longer can; then try the heavier dumbbell again.

## NOTES ON PHASE 2

You'll perform Phase 2 much like Phase 1, but here are some important notes and reminders to make sure you're on the right path.

- As with Phase 1, perform three workouts per week on nonconsecutive days, alternating Workout A and Workout B. Also like Phase 1, start each workout with a general warm-up, and perform warm-up sets for all exercises. Perform all sets for each exercise on its own before moving on to the next one in the workout.

- Record your workouts! Keep a logbook to track your workouts: weight used, reps performed, and any notes for that day's workout.

- The one thing that will change with Phase 2 is the rest periods between sets—they'll increase as you progress into the program and handle heavier weights. You may start out resting ninety seconds between sets, but that may increase to two to three minutes, especially for squats and deadlifts, since they can handle a lot of weight. Remember to rest as long as needed to put full effort into the next set.

- If necessary, you can start with cable pull-downs instead of chin-ups. Move to assisted chin-ups when possible.

- If you're not comfortable performing the bench press, or you'd like to progress to performing traditional push-ups on the ground, you can replace the bench press in Phase 2 with push-ups from Phase 1. Once you're able to perform 4x7 (four sets, seven reps) with push-ups, however, move on to the bench press. Push-ups are awkward to load with additional resistance.

- With Workout B, you have the option to alternate deadlifts and RDLs after following the program for at least eight weeks. Some trainees, after following the program for a couple of months, find deadlifting at that frequency can be a bit too much to recover from. If you experience the same thing, you can alternate deadlifts and RDLs each time you perform Workout B.

- You'll be able to stay on Phase 2 for several months, because these exercises allow for much greater loading potential than those in Phase 1. If you follow instructions and use fractional plates, at a minimum you should be able to continue making progress for at least sixteen weeks, but likely closer to twenty before something needs to change (depending on your strength training experience).

- The double-progression method (start at the low end of the provided rep range and stick with that weight until you reach the high end of the rep range for all sets, and then in the next workout add a little weight and start back at the low end) plus the loading potential of these exercises means lots of strength to build. Some of the exercises have different rep ranges, but the same guideline applies. The goal remains the same every time you repeat a workout: Do a little better than last time. Either perform one extra rep per set, or if you reached the high end of the rep range for all sets the previous workout, add a bit of weight and start back at the low end. Remember, in Phase 2 different exercises use different rep ranges. Look closely!

- Use fractional plates! You can buy them or make your own by getting two-inch washers at a hardware store, weighing them out, and gluing them together. These will get used soon, especially for the bench press and barbell press, because you can't handle as much weight on those exercises as you can for squats and deadlifts. By only adding one pound to the bar instead of five pounds (which is typically the lowest option at most gyms, since two-and-a-half-pound plates are the lightest available), you'll be able to make progress for much longer. That way you can keep getting stronger and milk out the greatest strength gains. Get, or make, a set of one-quarter, one-half, three-quarter, and one-pound fractional plates. Don't underestimate how incredibly useful these can be! You'll start using them within the first two months for the bench press and barbell press. Note: Making your own is much cheaper than buying a set.

- Once you've followed Phase 2 for about twelve weeks, you may want to take an "easy week" for extra recovery. For one week (a total of three workouts) reduce the weights 15–20 percent and stick to the low end of the provided rep ranges. Take this time to focus on exercise form. Then the next week, repeat the previous week's workout performance from the week prior to the "easy week," and keep progressing from there. You can perform an easy week every eight to twelve weeks.

- Several months into Phase 2, you may find it increasingly difficult to use the same weight for all work sets, or you may struggle to complete the same number of reps each set. If this happens, you can perform one top set with the heaviest weight you can use, and then take off about 10 percent for the remaining sets. For example, if you deadlift 205 pounds for five reps, but doing more than one set with that weight is extremely difficult, perform the first work set with 205 pounds for five to six reps. Then strip off 10 percent of the weight, and perform the last three work sets with 185 pounds for five to six reps. Once you reach the high end of the rep range for the first work set, add weight the following workout. You'll have to adjust the other sets too.

## HOW TO KEEP MAKING PROGRESS WITH PHASE 2

You should be able to make progress with Phase 2 for at least sixteen to twenty weeks (especially if you use fractional plates). But what should you do if you stall out and can no longer make progress on most exercises? You have several great options.

### OPTION A
If you can no longer add weight or perform more reps for most

exercises in Phase 2, the simplest way to continue making progress is to lower the rep range. Here's the original Phase 2 program.

Workout A:
   1. Squat
   2. Bench press
   3. Chin-up/pull-down: 4x5-7 reps for all exercises

Workout B:
   1. Deadlift/RDL: 4x5-6
   2. Standing barbell press: 4x5-7
   3. One-arm dumbbell row: 4x7-12

You can continue using the double-progression method with a lower rep range.

Workout A:
   1. Squat
   2. Bench press
   3. Chin-up/pull-down: 6x3-5 (6 sets, 3-5 reps) for all exercises

Workout B:
   1. Deadlift/RDL: 6x3-4
   2. Standing barbell press: 6x3-5
   3. One-arm dumbbell row: 5x5-8

The lower rep ranges will allow you to keep adding weight and getting stronger. And, yes, lifting even heavier weights is safe if you use proper form and weights you can confidently handle.

Wondering how you'll know if the weights you're using are too heavy? If you have to grunt, scream, and grind a rep to complete it—or feel like an eye is about to bulge out of its socket—then, yes, the weight is probably too heavy. Challenge yourself, yes, but use a weight you can control at all times, and don't attempt a rep you're not confident you can complete properly. Remember: Heavier weights are safe if you use proper form and maintain control at all times.

## OPTION B

If you have zero interest in lifting heavier, another option is to use lighter weights and perform higher reps. Here's how you can change the workouts from Phase 2 to fit this option:

Workout A:
1. Squat
2. Bench press
3. Chin-up/pull-down: 3x10-12 for all exercises

Workout B:
1. Deadlift/RDL
2. Standing barbell press
3. One-arm dumbbell row: 3x10-12 for all exercises

## OPTION C

And, finally, if you crave exercise variety, swap out the exercises in Phase 2 for different variations. Here's an example:

Workout A:

    1. Front squats

    2. Close grip bench press

    3. Pull-ups: 4x5-7 for all exercises

Workout B:

    1. Sumo deadlifts/RDLs: 4x5-6

    2. One-arm dumbbell push press: 4x5-7

    3. Chest supported dumbbell row: 4x8-12

That easily provides many months of training with the new variations. Once you stall out again, you can go back to the original Phase 2 program.

## WHAT TO WATCH OUT FOR

You have Phases 1 and 2 and know exactly what to do and how to progress, but here's some additional information, and helpful tips, to help you along your journey.

### FATIGUE IS NOT THE INDICATOR OF A SUCCESSFUL WORKOUT

If you're used to thinking of workout success as leaving the gym drained and depleted, your first few sessions are going to take some getting used to. You may find yourself thinking, "Wait...how am I leaving the gym with more energy than when I walked in? Did I do something wrong?"

The mentality that you must finish every workout utterly exhausted or you didn't go hard enough permeates health and fitness. There are workout programs and group classes that are about nothing more than burning as many calories as possible, and they glorify exhaustion and completing a workout feeling nauseated.

Likewise, women are encouraged to chase soreness. This feeling tells them they worked hard, that they did something good, because it's with them all day. "I can really feel yesterday's workout, so I know it's working."

Fatigue and muscle soreness are not badges of honor, and they're not the indicators of a successful workout. Sure, you will complete some workouts more tired than others, but you should not feel depleted at the end of most of them. Some muscle soreness is very likely during the first few weeks of Phases 1 and 2, but achieving it should never be a goal.

How then can you know if you had a successful workout? It all comes back to the logbook. Did you do better than last time? That means doing more reps with the same weight, or adding weight. Initially it could also mean improving exercise technique, too.

Improving your performance in some small way is what matters most—it's a simple, effective goal. A successful strength training workout is about getting a little stronger, not beating yourself into the ground.

## LIFT LIKE A GIRL IN REAL LIFE

"I cannot tell you how much happier I am now when the measure of my success is in a *positive* direction (e.g., how much weight I can lift this week) instead of a negative (e.g., weight on the scale). That coupled with the fact that I don't stress about food anymore, only train three times a week, and have plenty of time for family and enjoying other activities. I feel *so blessed* to have found your website and programs!"

Here are a few other things to look out for:

## LEARN TO EMBRACE THE SUCK

The longer you strength train, the more great workouts you will have and training milestones you'll crush. But it also means you'll have more workouts that flat out suck too. That's just the law of averages. This is an inevitable reality. You'll get information in the next chapter about bad workouts and how to work with them instead of against them. For now, though, know that you must embrace the suck—it comes with the territory. Don't get discouraged, and don't extrapolate from the situation (e.g., "I couldn't improve my performance in today's workout, so that means I failed").

Sometimes progress is just about showing up. Your body doesn't care that you want to add five pounds to your deadlift today. It may be tired from yesterday's activities and won't perform the way you want it to. Bad workouts will happen—just accept that fact now so you can look at it objectively.

## DON'T ADD EXTRA WORKOUTS

The exercises used in the programs were chosen for a reason: to deliver great results in the most efficient way possible. One of the best ways to screw up the program is to add a bunch of workouts on top of it. Occasionally I'll receive a not-so-nice email saying, "Nia, your program isn't working. And you suck."

But when I ask them to describe their week, it turns out they've been running on the treadmill for an hour after strength training, or doing HIIT classes on what should be off days, or they perform several extra exercises at the end of each workout.

They do too much, and it compromises their results.

More is not always better, especially with strength training. Quality, if you recall, trumps quantity. You're better off putting full effort and focus into the provided workouts instead of piling on additional exercises and workouts because you think that will lead to quicker, more noticeable results. Strength training—lifting weights and getting stronger—is one part of the equation. You must also *recover* from those things to actually reap the benefits they provide.

If you're used to performing workouts that have you moving at a rapid pace, or if you pile on lots of exercises in a single workout, this will be a shock to you. Resist the temptation to stack up your week with a bunch of other fitness activities and workouts. Commit to this strength training process and see where it gets you. If something else worked better, then I'd be telling you to do it.

## WHAT ABOUT CARDIO?

Worried about getting enough aerobic activity in your life? This is what you should do: Perform three strength training workouts per week on nonconsecutive days, as provided in Phases 1 and 2, and improve your performance each time you repeat a workout. That matters most. In addition to that, walk frequently, and play when possible.

If you have a job or lifestyle that keeps you sitting or

inactive most of the day, walking frequently is a great way to get in low-impact movement. If you have a very active, manual-labor job, this isn't as important for you. You can accomplish extra cardio by taking walks and following the common recommendations to take the stairs instead of elevator, park in the back of the parking lot, etc.

Beyond that, participate in physical activities you enjoy. Maybe you love a group Zumba class or a morning yoga routine. If you love those activities, keep doing them. Doing what makes you feel great, what you enjoy, is always good. Maybe you despise structured exercise but like being active in nature hiking, skiing, biking, and so on. Do it.

If there's a physical activity that brings you enjoyment and excitement, you should do it. But see, there's a difference between doing something for pure pleasure, and doing it because you think you have to.

On the days you don't strength train, move your body in fun, enjoyable ways (or simply walk) for about thirty to sixty minutes. This isn't a hard-and-fast part of the program—the main point here is that movement is good for your body (especially if you have a sedentary job). Those thirty to sixty minutes can be broken up too: It can be a twenty-minute dog walk in the morning and a twenty-minute yoga practice at night. Just keep it fun, simple, and not too intense.

Lighten up on the cardio for a while and focus on having fun and getting stronger.

Rule of thumb: Perform three strength training sessions per week, and move your body in some way (walking, participating in a physically active/enjoyable hobby) on days you don't strength train for thirty to sixty minutes (this can be broken up into chunks throughout the day).

## HOW TO HANDLE GYM INTIMIDATION

If you're joining a gym or going to enter the free weight area for the first time, it can be intimidating, especially depending on the culture of your local facility. If the free weight area is filled with grunting men who frequently let protein-shake-fueled farts fly with reckless abandon, it may not be the most welcoming environment.

Whether you're self-conscious about looking silly while learning the exercises, trying something new for the first time, or having to share equipment, or you feel like everyone will be watching you, it's normal. But you can shake this feeling and replace it with confidence. It just takes practice and fortitude.

If you're intimidated to enter the free weight area, there are a few things you can do. First, look at the big picture and what truly matters; you're in there to get stronger and become the best version of yourself. What other people think is irrelevant (recall our discussion in a previous chapter about internal vs. external motivation?). Just get back there, and get the first workout completed. Take your time if you must to learn proper form—you're doing this for you.

Second, get yourself in a zone, and ignore what's going on around you. Listening to your favorite music can be extremely helpful. This way you drown out the grunting and flatulence sounds around you and can focus on what you're there to accomplish.

Third, recruit a friend to go through the program with you. This way you can watch each other performing the exercises and provide cues if needed. For instance, you may notice that when your friend deadlifts she allows the bar to get out over her toes. You could cue her by saying, "Keep the bar over the mid-foot." Having a friend is great for camaraderie and accountability, and it's a great option if you like working out with someone.

> The journey of a thousand miles begins with a single step.
> —Lao Tzu

Remember, what everyone else is doing is irrelevant. You're there to become a better version of yourself. You're there to challenge yourself in a fun, empowering way. The first step is often the hardest. Just show up. Start going through the routine, and it'll become much easier. Yes, there is a learning curve to strength training. It is a skill, but it's a skill just like anything else you've had to learn in life.

A client shared with me that her gym was doing some remodeling, so there were workers in hard hats around during her workout. She said it bothered her at first, but then she remembered why she was there—in her words, "To kick ass." And that's exactly what she did. She didn't let the stares of construction workers get in the way of her plan to have a great workout.

## TIME TO LIFT

The strength training programs in this chapter give you a positive, empowering, performance-focused goal that let you discover the incredible things your body can do and help you to unleash your strength and reap the multitude of benefits that come with it. The programs allow you to reveal what you're capable of, and leave you wanting to do even more. Each workout leads you in a rewarding direction, toward greater physical strength, ability, confidence, and health. And, as you'll experience, each workout is its own reward, a reward for being alive, capable, and eager for more.

The programs are also meant to be enjoyable. Imagine walking into the gym with excitement, thinking, "Hell yes, I get to do better than last time. It's time to add five pounds to my squat and beat my previous performance."

## LIFT LIKE A GIRL IN REAL LIFE

"Here are some changes I've noticed as I celebrate one year of lifting:

- A friend who hadn't seen me in a while told me I looked amazing.
- My weight is down five pounds.
- I'm developing muscle definition.
- I can lift heavier weights.
- My everyday life is easier.
- Running no longer bothers my knees or hips.
- A new coworker was shocked upon learning my actual age—forty-eight.
- Other fun activities are easier: biking, kayaking, hiking, yoga.
- A coworker accused me of aging backward; she now calls me 'Benjamin Button.'
- A much younger friend told me she hopes she looks like me when she's forty-eight."

That's what I want you to experience with the strength training programs. Screw burning calories or getting as tired as possible or chasing soreness or performing as many exercises as you can cram in a forty-five-minute window. I want you to walk in the gym doors thinking how awesome it's going to be to deadlift two hundred pounds for the first time, or to add two pounds to the barbell press.

This is a journey that, the longer you're on it, the more

rewarding it will be. Get started immediately, and trust the process. Commit to Phase 1 for several weeks (four if you're not new to strength training; upwards of twelve if you are new), and then commit to Phase 2 for several months. Once you put in the work and experience the mental and physical benefits for yourself, I won't have to convince you of it anymore.

These workout programs won't make you a *new* you— they'll make you *more* of you.

The next several months are going to pass regardless of what you do, or don't do. Wouldn't you like to see what you're capable of achieving in that time and make the most of it?

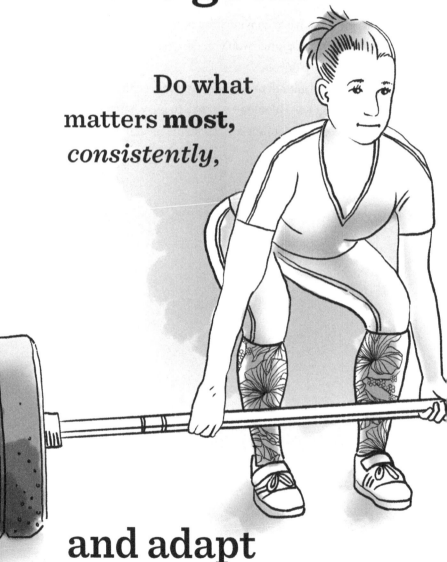

# Perfection *isn't* the goal.

Do what matters **most**, *consistently*,

and adapt when *necessary*.

# CHAPTER 5

# Perseverance, Not Perfection

The deadlift was naturally my strongest barbell exercise. When I committed to getting stronger, that lift kept going up and up, and I hatched a lofty goal: pull a triple-bodyweight deadlift.

At my peak strength, I was only forty-five pounds away from that goal. It sounded so awesome, and felt so attainable. My brain was repeating the words through every workout, "I've got to get there. I've got to pull 375. The sooner, the better."

I allowed my ego to take over my brain, and I kept pushing my workouts extremely hard. Too hard. I forced myself to improve my performance to the greatest possible extent every workout, even if that meant my form deteriorated; and I didn't let my body rest, no matter how desperately it needed it. Even days when weights that typically felt light had to be grinded off the floor, I kept pushing. "Screw it. I've got to get to that goal. I can't have an easy workout," is how I'd justify my actions.

I didn't realize it at the time, but this was the same obsessive, controlling mindset I previously applied to food, the mindset that led to disordered and binge eating. There's a lesson here: Don't trade one obsessive, controlling thing with another.

One week, I pulled three hundred pounds for three reps. The next week, I was determined to pull it for four reps. But from the moment I got started, everything felt horrible; it felt like the weights were glued to the floor. I didn't pull three hundred for four that day; I could only muster two reps. And I was pissed. I failed to improve my performance.

But I refused to let up, because my goal was within reach. I kept training hard, despite growing protests from my back to take a break, or at least to take it easy for a while. I trained through the discomfort, and then the pain. Eventually, I could no longer ignore the signals; what was acute pain turned into chronic SI joint pain. I couldn't squat anymore; I couldn't deadlift; I couldn't press a bar overhead. My training goals were derailed from an injury (a completely preventable injury, mind you). Even walking my dog hurt.

While recovering, I reflected over the experience. I didn't train myself the way I train clients. I never let clients push that hard for that long without cycling training volume and intensity. I never allowed their form to deteriorate, nor would I let them ignore important signals from their body. But I wasn't training myself with my brain—my ego took over. I wanted a goal, and I wanted it fast.

Goals are good, but actions are more important than the absolute goal. An obsessive, perfection-driven mindset shouldn't be applied to strength training. It prevents you from listening to your body, training intelligently, or seeing a broader image.

As I like to say to clients, "Live to lift another day." Many women quickly take to strength training, but their love for the challenge makes them want to hurry up and "get there," be it a huge deadlift, a bodyweight squat, or their first chin-up. But strength doesn't always happen on the timeline you want; strength training is a long-term game, and some goals will take longer to achieve. Having training goals provides motivation and excitement, but you need to be smart and improve your performance gradually and respect your body. Don't fight it when it says, "This isn't happening today."

## GOING TOO HARD

There are times when you may push too hard out of pure motivation to excel. At other times, though, going too hard means pushing yourself to keep up with what you feel is *normal* for you, or what you *should* do.

A client once told me that on a day between workouts, she spent the day helping her parents move. That meant lifting a ton of boxes, which she was able to do with ease, thanks to strength training. However, when she went into the gym the next day, she could tell her back was fatigued from the first warm-up set. She had, after all, spent the entire previous day hoisting and carrying heavy objects. Her response was stellar. She said, "I'm not deadlifting today. I'll do something else that doesn't put much strain on my back."

It was a smart choice, and she proceeded to improve her deadlift performance the next workout. You may be excited to deadlift five pounds more than last week, but if your body is fatigued, play it smart. Do something different for your workout that day, and give your body the recovery time it needs. If your body feels off, listen. It could be that you slept in an awkward position, or yesterday you tweaked a muscle without realizing it. If your body tells you it doesn't want to pull a deadlift personal record today, respect it. Either do a different exercise, or use less weight and focus on your form.

> It's important to improve your performance when possible, but some workouts it just won't happen. If you're fatigued or didn't sleep well the night before, lower the weights and focus on exercise technique. You can still have a productive workout without performing more reps than last time or adding more weight.

Strength training will hopefully become a powerful part of your life, but it should never *become* your life. In retrospect, that's what happened to me for a while, and ultimately led to my injury. People—my clients, my online community, my friends—knew me as the woman who likes to deadlift heavy stuff. I talked all the time about how much I loved it, how empowering it was, how it was instrumental in helping me appreciate my body for what it could do. But I didn't realize how much I had my identity wrapped up in that ability, until I couldn't deadlift anymore.

"What *can* I do?" was the only question worth asking when the goal I had was put on hold, and I couldn't do the lifts I enjoyed. Initially, I got a little depressed. Herein lies the problem: There's just as much danger in tying your value to some ability as tying it to some physical feature. There's always the possibility that, at some point, those things may be temporarily or permanently taken away from you.

The last thing I want is for *Lift Like a Girl* to become another cult-like methodology where a workout style becomes someone's whole reason for being. Make this part of your life, not something that defines who you are as a human.

After several weeks of being upset about my slowly healing back pain, I realized I was being stupid. I was upset over not being able to deadlift heavy, when that truly was not a big problem—it wasn't a life-threatening or life-altering change. Instead of obsessing over what I couldn't do, I committed to focusing on the abundance of exercises I could do, and to improve my performance with those exercises while my back healed. That way, I could continue to get stronger and train hard with purpose, and have fun while healing.

You may have read that story and immediately had your fear of getting hurt from strength training justified. Strength training is safe. Learn and use proper form; never sacrifice proper form for more weight or to squeeze out an extra rep. Listen to your body, and take it easy if you're worn out from a chaotic week. And don't let your ego take control because you're obsessing over a goal that is best achieved slowly. I got greedy, I stopped training intelligently, and that's why I got injured. Again, this is something I *never* let, or would let, a client do. But I wasn't looking at my training objectively like I do a client's.

More often, injuries occur outside the gym. I've worked with individuals who sustained an injury at work, during a hobby, or from tripping over their kid's toys and then had to wear a sling or a brace. In all but the most extreme cases (or if told otherwise from a physical therapist or doctor), I'll tell them to come for their training session anyway. No, they're not going to be deadlifting or squatting with a barbell on their backs; we focus on what they *can* do. It may mean using mostly machines or training the non-injured side, but they can still train, with a purpose, while they're healing.

Setbacks of some kind are inevitable, because life happens. Even if you don't get injured, you're going to get sick at some point and have to miss a week of workouts, or you'll vacation in a place where there's no gym, or a family emergency may take up all your time.

How do you get back into your workouts if you miss a week from illness, a vacation, or something else taking priority? If you just missed a week, reduce the weights about 10 percent and work back up to the weights you were using before the layoff. If you missed two weeks or more, take off about 20 percent and even start back with just two or three sets per exercise so you don't get too sore.

Sometimes life delivers situations that are more important than getting in a workout. Instead of getting upset about all the things you can't do, focus on the things you can do.

Having to take time off from my favorite barbell exercises gave me the opportunity to focus on other exercises I'd otherwise ignore. I ended up doing a lot of bodyweight exercises, because that's what felt best at the time, and I progressed to performing handstand push-ups for the first time. Focusing on what I could do, and getting better at it, was fun and motivating in a pleasantly unexpected way.

Bottom line, you never know what you can discover about your body, or a situation, when you find a way to make the most out of what you have.

## KEEP THE EGO OUT OF IT

Once I'd recovered from the injury, though, I had a new problem. Every time I added deadlifts back into my training, I would get stupid again. Instead of easing back into it slowly, intelligently—like I would make my clients do, but was too egotistical to do myself—I threw too much weight on the bar too fast. I remember thinking, "I am not going to just deadlift 135 pounds. I'm used to pulling 250 like it's a stack of cupcakes." Each time I did that, I would aggravate the injury. Frustrated, I decided to abandon deadlifting for a while. It was too fraught for me.

> Don't let your ego get in the way of smart training. If you're coming back after an injury, ease into training. You don't need to use as much weight as possible from the beginning. This isn't a race; there's no prize for adding weight fast. Build up gradually, diligently. Not only will you return to previous strength levels, you'll surpass them.

I avoided deadlifts until I was able to approach my training like I do my clients' programs—intelligently and void of ego. I admitted up front, before even touching the bar, that I was going to start back extremely easy. If that meant I'd be starting with sixty-five pounds, so be it. The goal was to deadlift pain-free, so the weight on the bar didn't matter. I started deadlifting with light weights, and committed to adding just five pounds each workout. My body could have easily handled increases of ten and even twenty pounds initially, but I stayed focused on the end game. Getting strong again was the goal, but there was no hard timeline to get there.

This happens with clients who complained about previously experiencing pain from squats or deadlifts. We would train those exercises, but at a much lighter weight than they were used to. They focused on using proper form on every rep, and gradually, a little weight was added to the bar each workout. They eventually returned to using previous weights, and then surpassing them, pain-free.

Clients routinely say that getting started wasn't the hardest part of their health and fitness regimen. It was if they had an unexpected break—they said getting started *again* was actually harder, because they lost some of the results they worked so hard to achieve.

When this happens, your best move is to shove the ego aside and just get going again. Even if you have to start out with less weight, do it. Rushing never works out well, but if you're patient and take the time to get back to where you were, you'll end up breaking through previous bests and continue going forward.

## BAD WORKOUTS HAPPEN

When you're new to strength training and don't have a lot of physical strength, you're not going to have a bad workout. But once you're stronger and more experienced, it's a fact that bad workouts are inevitable. The longer you do something, the more good days and bad days you're going to experience. It's part of the process.

These bad workouts can have any number of causes. Maybe you didn't sleep well the night before. Maybe you played extra hard with your kids over the weekend. Heck, there will be days you go into the gym feeling energetic and fantastic, but for some reason, everything, starting with your warm-up, feels sluggish and heavy.

The solution to bad workouts is to first "embrace the suck," as I like to call it. You can get pissed about it, force yourself to train hard anyway (despite your body giving you the proverbial middle finger), and risk digging yourself into a hole that takes longer to get out of than if you just took it easy that one workout. Or you can acknowledge that there will be days when your body isn't going to do what you want it to. Your body doesn't care what your workout log says you're supposed to do today, and it won't always cooperate.

Don't get emotional about your workouts. If you're going through the warm-ups and it feels like you're moving through quicksand, remind yourself to embrace the suck, and modify the workout to a point that feels safe and comfortable for your body that day. I recommend taking the weight down about 10 percent from what you did last time, and going through the exercise with extra focus on technique.

Another option is to cut the workout in half; this works great for days when you're low on energy. Where the workouts in Phases 1 and 2 call for four sets, just do two. Do your best with those two sets, focus on the form and quality of the movement, and then go home and let your body recover.

Getting stronger by improving your performance a little each time is imperative to achieving results. But forcing yourself when your body has other plans isn't a great idea. On the days when the weights feel heavier than usual even after repeating the first warm-up set or two, make the most out of what you can do safely and comfortably, and live to lift another day. One bad workout won't have a negative effect on your health, physique, or performance. Forcing yourself to grind through multiple ones in a row, however, can.

Our bodies can only handle so much stress. If you have an important work project that's demanding longer hours, or you've got personal stuff going on that puts your life at a high stress level, guess what? Your body may not have the resources to work out at the same level as usual. In this situation, you're better off not going 100 percent and crushing your workouts and chasing new records. Balance out the stress in your life by performing abbreviated workouts (two sets instead of four) or taking some weight off the bar until the additional stress wanes. Otherwise, what should be a way to build you up may burn you out.

## WHAT TO DO WHEN YOU OVERINDULGE

Sometimes, what was meant to be a meal of enjoying your favorite food turns into a weekend, which can turn into a week or more, of less-than-ideal food and drink choices.

Let's say you went on a trip with family or friends for the weekend, and you ate (and drank) much more than usual. In addition, you weren't in a place where you could sneak off for a workout. When you get home, you're not feeling as great as you were when you left. And you feel guilty for overdoing it.

We've all been in this position before, and we'll experience it again. Many women, even after following the *Lift Like a Girl* program for months, find themselves experiencing a guilt reflex after a bout of overindulgence. It's hard to separate that "blergh" sensation from shame and disgust at ourselves.

Most of the time, I successfully practice the nutrition guidelines in the previous chapter. But I still overdo it on occasion. I've eaten an entire small pizza and then, later in the day, followed it with a pint of ice cream. I've blasted through a sleeve of Girl Scout cookies when I planned on only eating a few. This is why I advise most people, myself included, to not eat foods directly from the package/container! I've also had too many handfuls of chips, candy, and other not-super-healthy foods at social gatherings.

During my obsessive, disordered eating days I'd beat myself up for those experiences: "I screwed up. How many calories was that? I better do an extra workout tomorrow." But now, my response is much different, "Well, that wasn't the best food choice I've ever made." And then I move on with my life and get back to the simple nutrition principles.

I know I'm not going to quit moving my body in ways that make me strong and powerful. I know that one day of eating more than I planned isn't going to harm me if I practice sound principles on a regular basis. The solution is to take emotion out of those choices; don't allow them to define you. It happened, you enjoyed it, and now it's a new day.

As discussed in chapter 2, what you say to yourself in those moments is crucial. Yes, you need to make smart choices about what you eat and how much you eat, but you also need to change the stories you tell yourself.

A favorite quote on this topic comes from the Stoic philosopher Epictetus: "Men are disturbed not by things, but by the views which they take of them."

This idea resonated so deeply that even centuries later, Shakespeare would take this very viewpoint from Epictetus and put it into one of his most iconic plays, *Hamlet:* "There's nothing good or bad, but thinking makes it so."

Ruminate on that for a moment, and how it can apply to something like overindulging.

When you eat a whole pizza and chase it with a pint of ice cream, you are the only one who gets to decide if that's good or bad…or neither. Don't think of yourself as a success or failure depending on what you eat from one day to the next. What really matters is what you do most of the time. And most of the time you will be choosing nutrient-dense, minimally processed foods that make you feel awesome.

## LIFT LIKE A GIRL IN REAL LIFE

"Today felt *fantastic*. There was a moment around rep three of set three of sumo deadlifts when I felt like I could lift the world. The shame voice is currently cowering in a corner. The weight I pulled/pushed around made me feel like a hero."

With both sides of health and fitness—strength training and nutrition—have compassion on yourself when things don't go as planned. You're human. You're fallible. This is why perfection is not your standard. Most people overeat at Thanksgiving dinner. It's typical to get lazy on vacation, or have a few too many tasty foods you don't get at home. It happens. When it does, don't assign a good or bad label to the event. Just move past it.

Furthermore, don't hide from the fact that you enjoyed it! If you were sick and had to take a day off from working out, instead of beating yourself up for it, relish the time you spent on the couch watching your favorite show. If you overdid it on the pizza and ice cream or whatever, let yourself enjoy the hell out of it. Then return to your regular routine the next day and start kicking butt again.

## ADAPTATION: YOUR SECRET TO SUCCESS

If there ever was a secret to success, it's adaptation. People who adapt are the ones who will have long-term success. It goes back to the fact that nothing is perfect. You're not going to do every workout and improve your performance every time, and eat nothing but real food, and always get plenty of protein, for the rest of your life. Something will happen where the routine gets derailed—or obliterated entirely—because something else in your life takes priority over you going to the gym.

The people who are able to sustain the results they've earned, and keep achieving more, are the individuals who are able to adapt to the situations life brings their way.

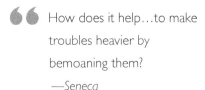 How does it help…to make troubles heavier by bemoaning them?
—*Seneca*

If you have a day (or span of time) when your gym time gets whittled down from sixty minutes to thirty, don't look at that and say, "I can only go for thirty minutes. There's no point. I'm not going to go at all." Instead, be willing to adapt: "Even if I can only do half of the workout, I'm still going to get in there and do the best I can in that time period."

The woman who injures her ankle playing with her kids may be tempted to skip the gym completely until it heals, but she knows adaptation to the situation is the best answer. That may mean doing upper-body exercises exclusively, but that's what she'll do until her injury is healed.

The woman who tweaked her back at work may not be able to deadlift heavy for several weeks, but instead of getting frustrated and quitting, she decides to use light weights and focus on her form until the pain is gone.

You will experience periods where you're short on time. You'll have to deal with an injury, or work around an old one. The equipment you need will be occupied. Something will happen. Instead of planning your fitness around perfection, how will you plan to adapt so you can keep moving forward?

Self-care is something that's often discussed among women today, but it's rarely practiced. It goes beyond treating yourself to a manicure or hot bath or a solo trip to the movie theater. It's about having compassion on ourselves when we need it. We beat ourselves up in a way we would never let someone do to our friends or family. We're much harder on ourselves than we ought to be.

Militantly demanding perfection might motivate you in the short term. But over the long term, it only has negative effects on your mind and body since endless perfection isn't possible.

## LIFT LIKE A GIRL IN REAL LIFE

"You've made me realize that being the best me isn't something I have to kill myself for. Because of that I can be awesome in all aspects of my life instead of just falling short on working out and feeling bad about it. I don't beat myself up anymore and, guess what, the weight is still coming off. My deadlift is 205 now, and I love lifting. It's not a love/hate relationship. Just love."

> Any man who does not think that what he has is more than ample, is an unhappy man, even if he is the master of the whole world.
>
> —*Epicurus*

If you start using cruel language in your self-talk, take a step back from the situation and look at it, objectively, as if it were happening to someone else. How would you respond to your friend or child or family member if she was going through the same situation you find yourself in? How would you encourage her to respond? You'd likely recommend a hefty dose of compassion and understanding.

In the same way that it's helpful to perform warm-up sets for strength training exercises to prepare your muscles, thinking ahead of time about how you'll respond to challenges and setbacks can make a tremendous difference when those scenarios happen.

"The man who has anticipated the coming of troubles takes away their power when they arrive," said Seneca, another Stoic philosopher. And it's true.

 Between stimulus and response there is a space. In that space is our power to choose our response.
—*Viktor Frankl*

When you finish this book, I hope you'll be excited and ready to strength train, get stronger, eat for health, and enjoy the whole damn journey. At the same time, I want you to have a realistic perspective and know that, at some point, something is going to happen that throws off your routine. It could be in a year, or it could be in a week.

Here's one way to arm yourself for future challenges: Think back to what usually gets you off track. What happened in the past that made you quit your health and fitness routine all together? Do you give up completely as soon as your routine is disrupted? Come up with a plan—write it down—that you can employ when that happens again.

If you expect challenges to arise and have a plan of action to employ when they emerge, you're going to be successful.

Know yourself, and prepare for common challenges. Then boldly face them instead of wishing they never happened. As the saying goes, hope for the best, but be prepared for the worst.

## MINDSET MANAGEMENT

It's a sad truth that our brains tend to fasten on the negative thought or feeling over the positive. Instead of focusing on the ten great workouts we did this month, we'll focus on the one or two we missed. We have to be intentional, and consistent, about reframing the stories we tell ourselves in a positive, empowering way.

This is where understanding the brain's negative feedback loop comes in handy. I first heard about this concept from writer Mark Manson (as he aptly calls it, the negative feedback loop from hell) in *The Subtle Art of Not Giving a F*ck*.

Let's say you overindulged over the weekend and feel guilty about it. I'm here telling you not to feel guilty for overindulging. Next thing you know, you'll feel guilty for feeling guilty about overindulging! You get stuck in a loop where everything you think about becomes fodder for that guilt.

Another tidbit gleaned from Manson is "the backwards law." As an example, the more you want to be skinnier, or leaner, or weigh less so you'll look better and be happy, the less likely you are to see yourself as beautiful, or actually be happy. Whenever you think about it, what you're really saying is, "I'm not attractive or happy now," and that decreases the likelihood you'll ever feel beautiful or happy despite any progress you make. That's a bleak perspective.

You can't let your happiness or self-worth be conditional. If you're not happy with your body right now, you may not be happy with it even once it looks better, whatever that means. If incessant dieting and frequent bouts of self-flagellation were a viable solution, wouldn't it have worked by now? If you're not happy with doing the best workout you can do each time you do it, you're never going to be happy with your performance or results.

You can, instead, choose to focus on actions that make you happy now. Learn to look at the big picture instead of lasering in on shortcomings or setbacks. If you missed a workout this week, don't fret over it. Instead, look at everything you've done the past several weeks. Instead of saying, "I missed a workout and screwed up," the better response is, "Wow, I've completed ten awesome workouts this month." That one missed workout doesn't matter as much as the fact that you've been consistent with your workouts over a long period of time.

Our brains naturally gravitate to the negative, so we must retrain them to focus on the positive. Transforming your mindset into a productive tool takes consistent, conscious practice. In the beginning, you'll have to work a little harder to retrain the way you think, to balance out a small negative with the overwhelming positive. But after a while, when your routine gets interrupted for whatever reason, you'll be able to move past it without wasting time and energy worrying about it.

Sticking with the common overindulging example, you can start telling yourself different stories. Instead of saying, "I overindulged," and then extrapolating, "Oh God. I screwed up again. I better do an extra workout," realize there's a space in between where you can choose how you're going to respond.

Let's start changing the stories we tell ourselves. Over-eating at our favorite restaurant is a blip on the radar. Maybe eating that much wasn't the best decision. Whatever. You enjoyed the hell out of every bite. Tomorrow, you're going to have a great workout that makes you feel good and makes you stronger.

This mental transformation doesn't happen overnight. Habits cannot be erased; they can only be replaced. I tell my clients—especially if they're deep in disordered eating habits and working out for punishment—it's important to be aware of the stories you tell yourself. It's not uncommon for a woman to start her day by getting on the scale in the morning and telling herself a depressing story about who she is. As she's putting on her clothes, she looks in the mirror and continues that self-defeating dialogue. When she eats a handful of M&M's at work, she repeats it again. By the end of the day, she could have told herself twenty soul-crushing stories about who she is, all of them reaffirming the negative habits she'd like to break.

The only way to break this pattern is to stop the negative conversation short. Find that space before the conversation escalates. What you say to yourself matters—it creates a snowball of momentum. Only you can decide whether it goes in a positive or negative direction. Put a space between the stimulus and your reaction, and choose how you're going to respond.

Let's say you wake up on Monday and realize you overslept. Normally, you cook a protein-rich, real-food breakfast, but today you don't have time. Instead you visit the drivethrough before getting on the freeway.

That breakfast doesn't help you feel as awesome as you normally do. At lunch, your blood sugar plummets, and you end up eating candy from the vending machine for a quick energy boost. By the end of the day, you feel lethargic. Instead of going to the gym like you usually do, you say, "Screw it," head home, and flip on the TV.

How would you respond to this day? Would you be able to respond with compassion?

Could you acknowledge that things did not go the way you wanted them to, but it's okay?

Could you say it wasn't your best day and not berate yourself, or would you think of yourself as a failure? Could you objectively learn from the situation to have a plan next time something similar happens?

That's the goal with this new story. Creating a new story lets you give yourself space to think through how and why things went the way they did, and to create a plan for achieving the outcome you want next time.

Upon examination, it's easy to see that things went wrong from the beginning. When you're rushed in the morning, you need a backup plan for a quick, healthy breakfast so you don't end up settling for fast food. An easy solution would be to have some premade smoothie ingredients put together and stored in the freezer so you can toss them in the blender and go.

Maybe you plan to go to the gym after work, but something consistently gets in the way. One of my clients told me she kept skipping her workouts, and as we looked for the main cause she said, "Well, I'm really hungry at the end of the day, and I just feel like going home and eating. I tell myself I'll go to the gym after I eat, but then I'm already home and ready to relax. Most of the time, I don't end up going."

That was an easy fix. If she was consistently hungry after

work, it meant her lunch was not holding her over through the workday. By bringing a protein-rich snack to work, she could tide herself over and even fuel her workout. She reported back that all it took was a protein shake and a piece of fruit at her desk to get her from work to the gym. She wasn't hungry, so she wasn't tempted to go home first and end up skipping her workout. Problem solved.

Sometimes a break in your routine is just an aberration. You were in a bad mood, you were extra tired, you were getting sick. But if you see that the routine break becomes a pattern—if you keep making poor food choices or keep skipping the gym—don't beat yourself up. Examine it objectively, and you'll discover the possible reasons why it's happening. That will give you the insight needed to find a positive solution that lets you start feeling awesome again.

Responding to situations with compassion allows you to find a pragmatic solution. You can't be the best version of yourself if you're constantly tearing yourself down. Change the stories you tell yourself, be compassionate, learn what you can, and have a plan going forward. Do your best to remove any emotion attached to your body, eating habits, and workouts, and find ways to do what makes you feel great.

## JUST SHOW UP

"I did not want to work out today at all. I procrastinated for hours. I talked myself into twenty minutes at the gym. I killed the workout today. Showing up works. This is a lesson my negative inner voice needed to learn."

This lesson came from an incredible coaching client, and

there's tremendous power in her statement. Sometimes you just need to show up and start doing the work, and the feelings will follow after. I've seen that happen in my own life too. I've had occasions when I didn't want to work out, and I didn't feel all that great, but I made myself do it anyway. I committed to just showing up and starting the process, and I was shocked that I ended up having a phenomenal workout. I finished feeling better than when I started.

### LIFT LIKE A GIRL IN REAL LIFE

"Proud of myself this week…I totally *do not feel like* working out (slammed with multiple deadlines at work), and I've done it anyway. It's the bare minimum warm-up, the lifting, and the cool-down, but I *went* and overcame the Don't Wannas."

This is another benefit of warm-up sets. If you get to the gym and "just aren't feeling it" that day, at least go through a few warm-up sets for the first exercise. Start moving and see how it feels. More often than not, just getting started will trigger your brain to go ahead and do the rest of it. A lot of times, you find yourself suddenly enjoying it.

## PERSEVERE

Perseverance, not perfection, should be your motto.

There will be challenges. There may also be setbacks. There will be slip-ups. There will also be numerous victories.

Change the stories you tell yourself. Expect and prepare

for challenges; boldly face—*and adapt*—to them. Celebrate all victories, and respond to mistakes with compassion and a determination to learn from them. Don't demand perfection, but choose to persevere.

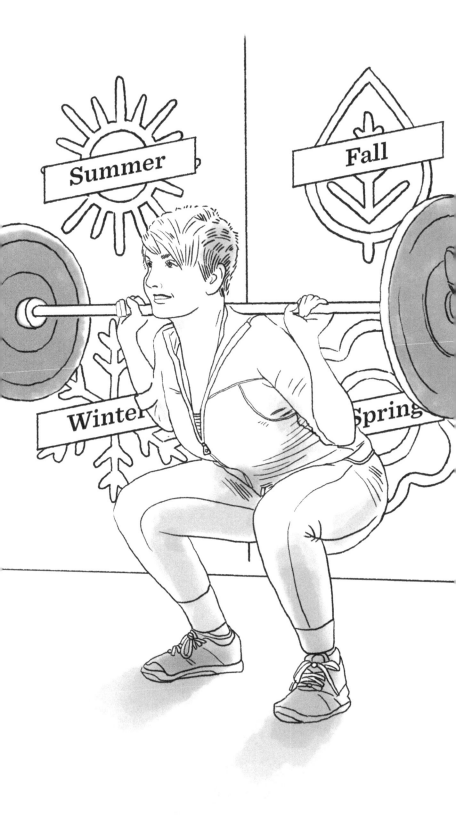

# CHAPTER 6

# A Lifestyle, Not a Fad

"I wanted to share a non-workout-related win. On Friday, I had to bury my Pa. I knew it was going to be a hard day. I got up early, went and killed my last workout for week three, walked out feeling really great. I drove three hours to the funeral. During the eulogy, my cousin couldn't speak on behalf of me and my cousins. I couldn't let him stand there alone with tears running down his face, so I got up to hold his hand and asked if he wanted me to read it. And I did. My legs were shaking, but I did it. I wouldn't have been able to do this three weeks ago, or even a week ago. I had confidence and got through what needed to be done. This program to me is more than just lifting; it's changed the way I think about me and what I can do, and not just in the gym."

This client's story is one of the most beautiful, powerful examples of how strength training is about more than getting strong in the gym.

I frequently extol the virtues of strength training, and relentlessly declare that it will make someone's entire life better.

Believe me, I understand how that can sound, well, stupid and hyperbolic. You have to experience it for yourself, because I can't prove it otherwise. But that's why I love that client's story. It reveals how getting strong in the gym makes a woman capable of things she wouldn't have been able to do before. The strength and grace and power in this woman, and all the women like her whom I've had the privilege to work with, is inspiring. It's *real-life* powerful.

## LIFT LIKE A GIRL IN REAL LIFE

"For anyone embarking on Nia's program for the first time, I just want to say keep at and don't *ever* give up or get discouraged! The end result is not nearly as important as the journey. You will discover so many amazing things about yourself, what incredible things your body *and* mind are truly capable of. There's an amazing feeling of empowerment, joy, confidence, and euphoria that is very hard to describe."

It's difficult to explain how squatting and deadlifting makes you strong, not just physically, but also mentally. Don't take my word for it; start doing it, and you'll experience it for yourself. Maybe it won't be in the same dramatic way this woman's story happened. Maybe it'll be in a smaller way only you can recognize. But the amazing truth, regardless of the circumstances, is how the strength shows up when you need it— how the strength will bleed into real-life events.

When you see what you're capable of doing in the gym— when you spend every week doing more reps and adding more weight to the bar—it will make you wonder, "What else am I capable of doing, above and beyond lifting weights?"

## LOOKING AHEAD

You're motivated, excited, and ready to put what you've read into practice. When you start, be sure to remember that this is *your* journey. It's essential that you don't compare it to anyone else's journey. As you jump in, don't look around and compare your starting point to another woman's. Commit to beginning from wherever you are right now, and moving forward at a consistent but comfortable pace.

This book is a guide to creating a lifestyle. You're not going to knock this program out in twelve weeks, get everything you can out of it, and then move on to something else. These are sustainable habits that are going to be part of your life and help you keep improving, hopefully forever.

For that to happen, though, it's important to ask yourself a question: Is this change I want to make something that I can see myself doing next week? What about five years from now?

This question is the premise behind why restrictive, rigid diets never work. If someone told me, "Hey, Nia, you can never eat ice cream again," I might say, "Okay," but I know damn well I absolutely will eat ice cream again. Probably that same day.

You can't avoid the foods you love forever, any more than you can do the same exhausting workout at peak capacity every day for the rest of your life. If you're going to make a change in your body, you must make sure it's based on changes you can maintain. That's the beauty of flexible, simple guidelines—they are, by definition, something you can do forever. They're not restrictive. There's nothing you have to categorically avoid. There's no declaration that you must be perfect. The guidelines can be molded to meet the specifics of your life and preferences.

The goal is to build health and fitness habits that fit into your life as a whole. For that to happen, your plan must be flexible, non-obsessive, and simple. You will do what delivers the most results, while leaving some leeway for other things. And you must enjoy it; otherwise you won't keep doing it. Commit to discovering what your body can do, and look at health and fitness as an exciting, evolving journey you get to take. It's more fun and motivating and creates a *more* mentality. By focusing on getting stronger, and growing your life to become more awesome, the workouts become something you get to do, not something you have to do.

Your journey will begin with a necessary learning curve, so be patient. Even the initial learning stage is fun, if you let it be. Strength training is, again, a growing opportunity for your mind as well as your muscles. Learning is fun. It's an opportunity to challenge yourself, to see what you're capable of.

## DEFINING YOUR GOAL

I foresee many women reading through the workouts in chapter 4 and panicking because there are only three exercises per workout. A lot of women will no doubt say, "Okay, well, I'm going to do extra exercises and barbell complexes and sprints at the end of each workout, and additional classes on the days off."

If that's you—if you're already thinking of adding more to the workouts—stop and ask yourself why. Why do you want to do more? Will those extra exercises/workouts/classes help you, and if so, how?

My guess is that you've been conditioned to think you have to do more. It's the outdated idea that if we're not exhausted and worn out at the end of a workout, we didn't do enough—that if some is good, more is certainly better.

If that's where you're coming from, don't add anything to the strength training programs. It's not going to help the way you think.

However, if you want to add something you enjoy doing, another activity you look forward to that makes your body feel great, then by all means, go do it. There's a big difference between doing something that makes you feel good, and lets you move your body in a way that's enjoyable, contrasted with doing something because you think you have to do more in order to burn off calories or punish yourself for what you ate.

It always comes back to understanding the mindset that is driving the actions you take.

Remember when cardio was seemingly the only workout option for women? It was simple, and it seemed easier to plod along on an elliptical machine for an hour than to put a loaded barbell on your back and squat. And that's not wrong. Having a barbell on your back demands focus; you can't zone out. Resisting a weight and maintaining proper form is challenging.

Over time, though, the slow, sustained cardio approach has morphed into workouts that are about "going hard" and getting as tired as possible. Exhaustion, soreness, fatigue—this is what women have been led to believe constitutes a successful workout.

This is why you will keep a logbook to record your workouts. It highlights the concrete improvements that really matter. If you improved your performance, your workout was successful. Period.

> To make the best of what is in our power, and take the rest as it occurs.
> —*Epictetus*

The logbook is also helpful to journal your way through the journey. You can write down notes about how you felt, what you focused on, and breakthroughs you experienced. Those little notes are powerful because you can look back at them to see how far you've come, which becomes especially helpful on days when you're feeling off or unmotivated.

Finally, don't be afraid to make small, temporary changes that help you toward your bigger goal. When I was breaking away from my obsessive eating habits and negative body image, I got rid of my scale, quit looking at myself in the gym mirrors, and even wore looser clothes for my workouts, so I couldn't hone in on the body parts I hated. That may seem like an extreme measure to take, but it's what I needed to do.

I knew it wasn't possible to quit hating myself immediately. I needed "blinders" that would let me see past my physical appearance and put my focus onto my physical performance. That allowed me to start having fun with my workouts, which made me want to keep getting stronger and doing better.

Gradually, that's what allowed me to start appreciating my body, because I was aware for the first time of what it could do and why that was so awesome and rewarding. That process helped me appreciate how my body looked physically through the discovery of what it was capable of doing.

## LIFT LIKE A GIRL
## IN REAL LIFE

"You are the only person who truly helps me focus on what is important. I believe in getting stronger, and if other parts of me change physically to keep up with that—that's awesome! Your approach helps me develop a more well-rounded sense of self, rather than focusing only on my superficial image. Mirrors no longer own me—I only care about how I feel in my own skin!"

"Spot reduction" is a myth. You can't control where your body sheds fat. However, strength training allows you to build your body. If you don't want the back of your arms to look droopy, building muscle will lift that area.

It's okay to do things differently from the other women you know, whether for a long time or just at the beginning. We've all had our own experiences that make us view ourselves and health and fitness the way we do, and we all need to take our own approaches to improving our view of ourselves.

I say again, this is your journey. Don't forget that. It will not look like mine or any other woman's. Take into account your previous exercise history, health and injury history, and your mindset at the present moment, and find your own way to make this process work for you.

# KNOW WHAT YOU CAN, AND CAN'T CONTROL

The Stoics use a metaphor of an archer that beautifully illustrates a healthy approach to fitness. An archer can control the arrow he selects, how he sets up his arrow, how he draws his bow, and his precise aim where he wants the arrow to pierce, and he can release at the right moment. But the second he lets go of the arrow, he can no longer influence the outcome of the arrow. Whether it hits the target or not is beyond his ability at that point. After he lets go, a burst of wind can knock the arrow off course, for example.

This demonstrates the glaring fallacy of absolute outcome-based goals (i.e., the bull's-eye).

The lesson is clear: Focus on the actions within your control. You can aim for the target and prefer to hit it, but demanding it is beyond your ability.

 *First tell yourself what kind of person you want to be, then do what you have to do.*

*—Epictetus*

A healthy lifestyle is about doing the best you can, with what you have, and understanding the difference between what you can control and what you can't control—and accepting it. That is why you must choose to focus on the actions (and thoughts) that make you feel like *more*, not less. More powerful, more awesome, more healthy.

So, what can you control? Your mindset and your actions. That's it. Despite what marketing and media say (and try to sell you), you can't completely control how your body will transform. You can't mimic a professional athlete's training regimen and expect to look like her. You can't control whether your body sheds fat from your thighs or upper arms first. You can influence the outcome, but you can't completely control it.

All you have control over is what you choose to do and think. This is true about everything in life, and it's inextricably tied to health and fitness.

Therefore, action-based goals are the answer. Choose to focus on what you can do—and thereby control—and not on the exact results you want to achieve. This is the difference between saying, "I *have* to lose belly fat and shrink my thighs," and choosing instead to say, "I'm going to perform three strength training workouts per week." It's the difference between saying, "I have to stop thinking about food all the time," and "I'm going to apply the simple nutrition guidelines, and I'll start with just one small change if I must."

You may want to lose the fat on your belly, but your body may shed the fat around your butt and thighs first. You can't select where it'll come off first; your body will.

Be the archer in the metaphor, and perform the actions within your realm of control. Strength train three days per week and improve your performance each time, start practicing the nutrition guidelines—and then let go. You can prefer to hit the target, but you can't command it to happen exactly how and when you want it to. You may miss the bull's-eye the first time because you encountered a setback (a gust of wind, in this example) beyond your control. Take aim, and try again.

# CELEBRATING WINS OF EVERY SIZE

Abolishing the quick-fix mentality can be a struggle initially. We tend to believe that once we figure out the right way to do something, we should see results, and we should see them quickly.

How can someone stay motivated to keep working out and eating well if progress seems to occur at a glacial pace?

The antidote is to find, and celebrate, the small wins. Did you go to the gym today? That's a small win. Did you take the time to learn correct technique for the exercises without letting what other people may think deter you? Another win. Did you find some new protein-packed snacks you enjoy and keep you energized? Did you embrace the moment between stimulus and response and choose not to respond critically for enjoying more cookies than you intended to? Win. Every action you take, no matter how small it seems, that leads you in the direction you want to go is grounds for celebration.

We typically gloss over the small, frequent wins because, let's face it, we're interested in radical transformations: building a certain figure, losing a specific amount of weight, achieving that first unassisted chin-up. And we're not happy until we get there.

Those big wins are worthwhile goals. But they shouldn't prevent us from appreciating the surplus of small wins we rack up along the way. After all, it's this accumulation of small wins that brings the big goal to fruition. Every workout should be a win, because you're moving your body, getting stronger, and doing something good for yourself. Combine that with implementing the nutrition guidelines, and that's an impressive list of wins. With each small win, you're reinforcing the actions that are going to lead you to a desirable outcome.

Along with celebrating physical wins, such as gym performance and nutrition, take the time to respond to the conversations you have with yourself. If you find yourself stopping the conversation short and refusing to tear yourself down, changing the story in a positive way, then that's a win that should be savored.

Appreciate yourself every time you do something good for you that builds you up. This is where journaling is handy. Whether it's in your workout logbook, in a hardcover notebook, or even on an app on your phone, write down those wins. Write down how you feel about them, and how you plan to replicate them.

Don't obsess over a particular long-term, distant goal. Instead, appreciate the actions you employ on a daily basis that lead you toward a desirable outcome. Gladly collect your small wins.

## THE WORKOUT *IS* THE REWARD

You won't finish every workout energized. Some days you're going to be tired. Some days you'll maybe even be exhausted if your workout was preceded by an overwhelming day at work. Most of the time, though, I encourage women to conclude a workout saying something to the effect of, "Hell yes. I just did that. My body is awesome."

I want her (and you!) to feel proud about what she did and accomplished. That mindset will serve you well, and it's preferable to something most women say, such as, "I feel like I'm going to vomit, but at least I worked hard enough to burn off the calories from last night's burger and fries."

Working out should feel good at a foundational level. It should make you better. It should be something you enjoy.

Be proud of what you do in the gym—allow a workout to be a reward in and of itself instead of seeing it as a chore ("Just ten more of these workouts, and I'm finally going to look better!") for a better outcome.

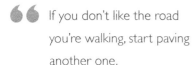

If you don't like the road you're walking, start paving another one.

—Dolly Parton

Let's abandon the flawed approach that says tons of exercises are necessary, that you must complete a workout extremely tired, and, if you do have energy left, you need to do intervals or some other high-intensity exercise to finish you off. Let's get strong, not tired. That means completing a workout saying, "I felt great today. I could've pushed a little harder, but that means next time I'll come back and do better than I did today." This creates a positive focus. Your actions have a purpose.

The *Lift Like a Girl* philosophy means making each workout its own reward. You do it because you're capable, because you're alive, because you're awesome, because it makes you more of the woman you want to be at home, at work, in life. We often take for granted our body's abilities, but working out should remind you how blessed you are to have a capable body that can do amazing things.

## FEEDING THE HABITS YOU WANT TO GROW

Today, I took a dose of medicine—my own flavor. I didn't feel like working out; plopping down in front of the TV was a more appealing option. But I was faced with a choice of which habit to feed, the habit of working out even though I didn't "feel like it," or the habit of skipping it.

What I tell clients, "The habit fed most often will be the one that wins long-term when challenges arise." When that advice popped into my mind, the choice was much easier: show up and do the work. It wasn't the best workout I've ever had, but I did it. And I was glad I did. No one regrets a workout.

Now, you could argue it was an easy decision for me to work out despite not wanting to, because I've been strength training for close to two decades. But I think of it this way: I've been strength training for almost two decades because I've regularly fed the habit of strength training, especially on the days I didn't "feel like it." I've successfully established a habit I can rely on when my brain has other ideas about what would be more fun. Because this habit is deeply ingrained, I'll be strength training for many more decades to come.

There will be days when you don't feel like working out, but show up and do the work anyway. There are exceptions. If you're sick, you may be better off resting or doing something easy like going for a walk. If you're on the brink of vomiting or have a fever, heavy deadlifts are the last thing you need to do. Rest, and get better.

We cannot choose our external circumstances, but we can always choose how we respond to them.

—*Epictetus*

If you're in the midst of an extremely stressful period, don't dig yourself deeper by piling on strenuous workouts. Easy workouts, with lighter weights, have their place and worth. If you're under more than normal stress, it could benefit you to perform fewer sets (two instead of four) or decrease the weights until things calm down. This way you're still feeding the habit of training, but don't risk adding so much stress it could be detrimental.

Our habits determine who we are, and what we will become. The habits that get created, and ultimately thrive and flourish, are the ones we regularly feed.

When you're faced with a similar situation, ask yourself: Which habit am I going to feed? Which habit do I want to still have ten years from now?

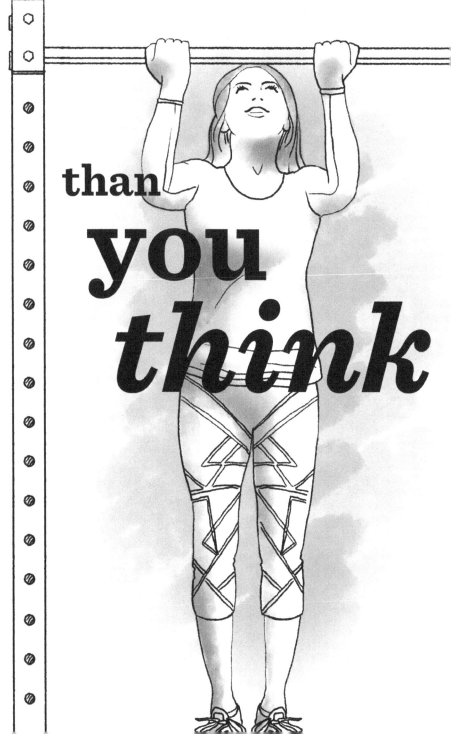

# CONCLUSION
# You're Stronger than You Think

Time for some shameless gloating—not about myself, but about my mom. My mom is amazing, so I'm going to share her badassery with you. Her family has an extensive history of breast cancer; it took one of her sisters. My mom was diligent about self-exams, mammograms, and had multiple biopsies that revealed a cause for concern. After conversations with her doctors, they decided it was in her best interest to get a prophylactic mastectomy.

Leading up to the surgery, my mom was determined to get as strong as she could. She wanted something positive to focus on, and she knew that further increasing her strength would help aid her recovery from the surgery.

After the mastectomy and reconstructive surgery, she was committed not only to regain her previous strength, but to surpass it. She wanted a goal to train for to keep her focused, so she planned to enter a powerlifting meet about six months after her discharge. She wanted to prove to herself that she could come back stronger than ever.

She trained intelligently and started out easy at first, avoiding exercises that could negatively affect the healing (namely, the bench press). Slowly she started doing more, and adding more weight. When she competed at the powerlifting meet, she didn't just lift—he beat some personal records.

The powerlifting meet wasn't just about setting personal records. It was something she said she wanted to do, to prove to herself that getting her breasts removed wasn't an obstacle she would let hold her back or affect her self-worth. She alone could decide what that meant and how it would affect her. Because she's a badass, she used it as an opportunity to become more.

## A GROWTH MINDSET IS THE KEY TO BEING MORE

True or false: You're smart, or you're not—either way, what you were born with is what you get.

Answering *True* signals a fixed mindset. This mindset says you're smart or talented, or you're not—you can't change it, because the abilities you were born with are as good as it'll get. People with this mindset might have said in school, "I can never learn this because I'm stupid."

Answering *False* indicates a growth mindset. This mindset says you can increase your knowledge, learn new skills, and improve your abilities. You may have to work brutally hard, but you can make progress. These are not innate traits, but learned abilities.

In *Mindset: The New Psychology of Success*, Carol Dweck explains and explores this topic in detail. According to her research, no matter where you're starting from, you can always grow. You're not stuck with what you were born with; you can improve.

There's another distinguishing trait between a growth mindset and a fixed mindset. Those who tend to exercise a fixed mindset view failure as proof of what they already believe. If they actually try to do something and fail, it reinforces their conviction that they will never succeed. They see failure as a defining event, proof of their unchangeable limitations.

On the other side, people with a growth mindset know improvement is possible. They can get smarter and learn new skills; they can improve their abilities. They know it may not come easily—they may have to work ferociously over a long period of time to see the success they want—but they know it's possible. When it comes to failure, individuals with a growth mindset view it as a valuable experience and learning opportunity—it's not an identity. They may try something and fail, but that experience doesn't define them. Instead they may say, "I tried this and it didn't work as I expected. What could I do to be better next time?"

In the realm of health and fitness, numerous women feel, after trying several diets and workout programs, that they're destined for failure. They believe that trying and failing makes them a failure.

The reality is that no past failure defines you, and neither will a future one. Improvement is possible, as long as you consistently put in the effort. Even if you weren't raised on healthy food, you can learn to eat well. Even if you've never been the least bit physically coordinated, you can learn to do new exercises. Even if you got made fun of in gym class, you can get stronger. Even if you tried dozens of other approaches in the past, this time can be different, in the best way possible.

I've worked with so many people who've been stuck in the same mindset for years. They think they can't change. They believe nature dealt them a bad hand. There's nothing more rewarding for them than finding out, after several weeks of consistent effort, that they can change.

I've had women tell me when we first started working together, "You don't understand how horrible my genetics are. You don't know how bad my family's health history is. You have no idea how hard it is for me to make any discernible progress."

After a compassionate discussion, my concluding response is, "You're right. That absolutely sucks for you. So what are you going to do about it?"

In this example, there are two options, and only one is good. Be a victim of your circumstances and continue to complain and be miserable and wallow in a fixed mindset that will never serve your best interests, or adopt a growth mindset, acknowledge the challenge in front of you, and choose to forge forward regardless. Even if you have to claw and scratch for it, significant progress is possible. The harder you have to work, the more rewarding it is to achieve, because you know damn well you earned it.

Another interesting factoid Dweck explains in her book is that it's possible to have a growth mindset in one area, but a fixed mindset in another. You may be confident that you can get smarter by studying and working hard, while at the same time believing that when it comes to your fitness, you're a prisoner of nature or nurture.

Need help forging, or strengthening, a growth mindset? Think about something in your life that you had to sweat and sacrifice to achieve. Something nobody would help you with, that you had to get out there and earn.

Maybe you're a single mom determined to raise your kids well.

Maybe you attended night school for years to complete your degree.

Maybe you saved up money, one tiny fraction of your paycheck at a time, to buy a house.

That same "bust your ass" ethic translates perfectly into health and fitness, if you want it badly enough. A woman may take years to build up to a bodyweight deadlift, but if she patiently takes her time and fights for it, she's going to achieve it.

These milestones we achieve are sweeter *because* of the hard work that goes into them. We can look back and say, "Hell yeah, I earned that victory. I counted every drop of sweat and blood and perseverance that went into it." The fight is what really allows you to appreciate your achievements. Things may not be easy, but that doesn't mean they're impossible.

Harness the power of a growth mindset.

## HERE'S WHAT'S NOT GOING TO HAPPEN

Even with good fitness information, people can have an idea that's unintentionally misleading. They assume that if they follow the advice, everything will be easy. Clever marketing shares the blame because they promise things like, "Get fast results easier than ever before!" And when it's not faster and easier than ever before, people feel as if something must be wrong with them.

I want you to close this book with a clear, accurate understanding of what happens next.

We're blessed to live in a time filled with medical advances, modern conveniences, free shipping with no minimum purchase required, animal videos so damn sweet it'll give you a cavity, and great opportunities to create the life we want. Unfortunately, our world no longer demands anything of us physically to survive. Inventions are constantly created to remove physical effort from our lives.

One of my pet peeves is seeing someone push a loaded shopping cart around a supermarket for an hour, unload everything from the cart into their car, and then refuse to push the empty cart fifteen feet into the cart rack in the parking lot. And, yes, I flash the stink-eye to the perpetrator.

That's how our society is, to a large degree. We try to shave effort out of our lives wherever possible. Our environment has conditioned us to avoid exerting ourselves.

Some fitness clubs aren't exempt from this "easier is better" mentality. They have tons of exercise machines. Why? Because it's easier to sit in a machine and move your body through the fixed, predetermined range of motion than to walk up to a barbell on the floor and use focus, balance, coordination, and mental fortitude to pick it up.

This isn't to say machines are worthless—if that's where you need to start to build confidence, or it's the only option while an injury heals, or it's the only available option, that's fine. But in this book, the goal with the strength training workouts is maximum efficiency—to develop the greatest qualities with the fewest mandatory exercises. Usually the efficient exercise is going to be the harder exercise. A squat will build total body strength, balance, coordination, and mental fortitude in a way a leg press simply cannot. Since you must control the barbell and your body movement in space as opposed to just pressing the platform on the leg press machine, it will be harder.

## THE UNCOMFORTABLE TRUTH

Many jobs nowadays are sedentary and don't have physical requirements. Combine that with the fact that we use tools like elevators, escalators, and cars so that we don't have to put forth physical exertion. I've had able-bodied neighbors who got in their car to drive to their mailbox, a mere thirty yards away. It explains why many people despise the feeling of having to resist a weight on their back when descending into a squat.

For most people, it's a foreign sensation to have to put forth effort, focus, and even a bit of strain to resist a weight pressing down on them, even if they can physically handle the demand safely. "I hate this feeling! Get me out of here!" is a response I've seen from people who visit a gym for the first time. Most of us go through life without having to face physical challenges with any frequency. We've been conditioned to react to physical demands as a bad thing.

But without challenge, there cannot be any growth. In

fact, the absence of challenge causes regression. You don't just stagnate; you go backward.

A growth mindset means viewing challenges in a new way—as an opportunity to become more. It may be uncomfortable, but like anything else, the more you practice it, the more you force yourself out of your comfort zone. Bit by bit, the easier it will become to face challenges.

Think of it this way: Going to the gym means choosing voluntarily to put yourself in an uncomfortable situation for the sake of becoming stronger. It's a place where you get to practice taking on challenges, so when life inevitably hurls an obstacle in your path that you didn't choose, you feel more prepared to face it.

I want you to be excited to begin your journey, but I won't sugarcoat the truth. There are books and resources readily available that will promise you easy, quick, immediately visible results. Because that's what people want to hear—we want to believe that's true.

But the uncomfortable truth is that it won't always be easy. You'll have tremendous periods of progress, but then you may stall for a bit. Your schedule may cooperate with your gym regimen, but chaos may ensue without warning. Nobody wants to hear that at times it will get tough, and they'll have to commit to overcome the challenge. But you need to know the truth so you can prepare for it.

Frankly, sugarcoated half-truths are condescending. Strong, badass women like you deserve to hear the truth and make your own choice about what to do with it. You have to begin this journey knowing there will be challenges, and even setbacks. But if you know from the beginning that it won't always be smooth and simple, those challenges are not going to divert you the way they would if you weren't expecting them. When they arrive, you'll be able to take on challenges with confidence, determination, and even excitement about where the process will take you.

Starting a new fitness program is like beginning a romantic relationship. You're excited, you're happy, you're drunk with infatuation. But once that newness starts to wane, that's when the work of cultivating a fruitful, strong, lasting relationship begins.

By this point, I hope you're excited to begin your strength training journey. In the first month, you'll progress quickly and feel incredible. But know that at some point in the future—it might be a month, it might be a year—there's going to come a moment when you will flirt with the idea of breaking up with strength training. You're going to ask, "Why do I put up with this? All it does is make me strain and sweat and work incredibly hard, and results are coming at a slower pace." You'll want to throw up the middle finger and dive face first into a gallon of ice cream.

Some people put their self-care on the back burner when life gets chaotic. They get loose with their food choices and stop working out. They take care of everything and everybody else first.

Some women will have to work harder than others for visible results, and they may feel as if they're not meeting their goals quick enough and wonder, "Why am I working this hard if results accrue so slowly?"

Others may simply fall prey to boredom. Even I go through this at times too—I've had moments when a barbell was the last thing I wanted to see, and I didn't want to write or mutter a word about nutrition or strength training. I wanted to blow up my computer, order pizza, and watch Netflix while my butt carved a permanent imprint in the couch.

Anything you do long enough—whether it's your job or a hobby or a relationship—is going to involve days when you're frustrated, bored, or distracted. It could only last for an hour, or it could extend over weeks. In those times, it's vital to recall the importance of this part of your life. What is the greater purpose of this? Why did you bring it into your life in the first place? That's what you must focus on to trudge through the swamp and emerge on the other side.

There's an expectation that fitness should always be simple, that you should never have to struggle with it. If it's not simple, some people think that either they or the program are defective. When I reveal that I go through periods when I don't love strength training, or that I struggle to make as much progress as I'd like, some people are shocked. Strength training isn't just my hobby; it's my job. But I remind myself why I do it and what I love about it, and I hold tight to the greater purpose to get through the slump.

Admittedly, I'll never stop strength training, because it's a deeply ingrained habit. It's part of who I am. It can be for you too. Eating well and strength training should be a lifelong habit, something you still do even if you're having a "screw it all" kind of day, because it's part of who you are.

Quitting shouldn't be a long-term option. You may

occasionally go a week or even a month without training because, hey, life happens. But it must be a habit, something you do not just because you love it, but because there's a greater purpose to it.

When you start eating and lifting the *Lift Like a Girl* way, it will become part of who you are, because you'll experience the invaluable difference it makes on your body, mind, and life. I believe this, because I've seen it happen more times than I could possibly count.

## IT'S UP TO YOU

You were challenged from the beginning of this book to shift your focus away from the appearance-obsessed, "it's all about fat loss" mentality plaguing women's health and fitness.

Women are becoming increasingly fed up with always thinking about, and trying to achieve, fat loss. And that's a good thing. You don't have to do it anymore. Screw fat loss and all the shrinking, blasting, whittling, and zapping that goes with it. Forget about everything that pressures you to be less, and unleash your awesome. You have the right to find out how good it feels to live for more.

Disregard the marketing and memes that feed the idea that the only fitness goal a woman can have is losing fat. Choose instead to focus on your performance; your physical form will follow your physical function. The way your body transforms from consistently practicing the nutrition principles and performing the workouts is largely determined by your genetics. A woman with wide hips will look radically different at her fittest than a woman with narrow hips and broad shoulders. How your body responds to progressive strength training will be unique to your body, so embrace it.

Strength training unlocks your individual potential for strength. This is largely untapped for most people. This is why it's a phenomenal tool to "unleash your awesome." If you're new to strength training or fitness in general, you're going to be amazed by what your body is capable of doing. It lets you get to know your body in a completely different way. Everybody will naturally excel at certain exercises because of their individual body shape and structure. Embrace the body you have to work with, appreciate it, and be proud of it.

As with any other endeavor, you'll get out of training what you put into it. The person who skips more workouts than she performs and doesn't challenge herself with an appropriate weight will achieve results that reflect this level of commitment. The woman who takes the time to learn proper exercise technique and performs the workouts consistently, while steadily improving her performance, will reap greater results: increased strength, better balance and coordination, increased confidence, and improved body composition.

My job is to equip women with the information and workouts needed to achieve the greatest results, in a way that fits their lives. But I'm not responsible for the lack of results they don't work for. Occasionally, some will come to me griping about their lackluster results, blaming the workout program. Upon examination of their actions for the past couple of months, the program wasn't the problem. They didn't perform the workouts as instructed; they didn't apply the nutrition guidelines consistently. At best, their consistency was sporadic. That's why the results were minimal.

Only you can implement the information that's been placed in your hands. Only you can do the work. I can't be there with you to make sure you're doing what needs to be done.

At the same time, don't hear what I'm not saying. "You'll get out of it what you put into it" isn't a license to seek faster results by depriving yourself and to feel as if you're sacrificing your livelihood. Some people assume that if doing some is good, more is always better. That's not what this book is about. Results come from consistently doing what matters most, and building an enjoyable, sustainable, flexible lifestyle. Show up, do the work, focus on the empowering benefits, disregard the massive amount of bullshit that plagues the health and fitness industry, keep your sights focused on what matters, celebrate your wins, and have fun.

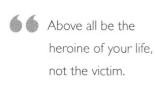

Above all be the
heroine of your life,
not the victim.

—*Nora Ephron*

The only journey worth traveling is the one that progressively leads you to being the best version of yourself. Most of what's in the health and fitness world is the antithesis to this goal.

If you're not becoming the best version of yourself, what the hell *are* you doing?

## REMEMBER WHO'S LOOKING AT YOU

What women do and say about health, fitness, and their bodies affects more people than themselves. If you look in the mirror and your five-year-old daughter hears you blurt out, "Oh my

God, I hate my thighs. I'm so fat," that will likely leave an impression on her if she hears it frequently.

If you engage in discussions with women about how you cheated on your diet and have to go burn off the calories or how you need to get serious and finally lose weight because that will make you happy, then you're adding fuel to the mentality that women are flawed and the only goal we can have with eating well and moving our bodies is to lose fat and look better.

We're social creatures, and we mimic the behavior and adopt the habits of those we spend the most time with. It would behoove us all to remember who's watching us, and to allow this to influence our words and behaviors. And it's never too late to change course.

Now let's revisit the above scenarios. The mom stands in front of the mirror while her five-year-old daughter looks on. She says, "These pants are getting a bit too snug. My strong thighs and butt have added muscle from those squats I've been crushing in the gym. Time to get some new clothes that fit my strong, awesome body."

The women at work moan about all the extra time they'll have to spend in the gym after enjoying birthday cake during lunch. They glance your direction for input and you say, "I'm not worried about it. It's just a piece of cake. I'll eat a protein-rich dinner and then go break a deadlift personal record tonight at the gym."

You can choose to show the young girls (and young boys) and women in your life that women can be strong, can be powerful, can choose for themselves, and don't need the approval of other people to make their worth any better. Just think of the measurable impact that could have on the world. Everything in our circumstances starts from within us. How we judge ourselves shapes the culture we live in.

Wouldn't you love to live in a world where moving your body was something everyone did because it feels amazing?

Where being physically strong is considered more important than being conventionally beautiful?

Where the choices you make and values you practice are prized as being beautiful more than winning the genetic jackpot?

Where nobody was compelled to revolve their eating habits around losing weight and fitting into a smaller pair of jeans?

You don't always know who is watching you. If you knew they were watching, what message would you want them to take away from what they see and hear? Seeing a woman deadlift heavy weights could be a foreign sight to a woman 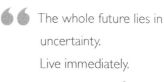 The whole future lies in uncertainty. Live immediately.

—*Seneca*

at your gym, but watching you may make her think, "Holy crap, look at her kicking ass. Maybe I should try it."

You never know who you can positively influence by what you do and say.

Don't be afraid to be your own heroine. There's nothing wrong with having role models—there are many people I revere, and I try to emulate the qualities I admire. But even more important is being able to define yourself on your own terms.

I've witnessed the women in my life go through

heart-wrenching trials, and they keep blazing forward. It's impressive and inspiring. They don't wait for someone to rescue them. They realize they are in control, and they are more than enough to meet the challenges life brings them. If you want something to change, you're better off taking action on your own than waiting for something to get better.

After you finish this book, I hope you're ready to start your empowering journey. But, please, don't wait for next month or Monday or (God forbid) New Year's Day. Don't put it off until life calms down or you have more time. There will never be a perfect time—as soon as one situation calms down, there's going to be another to replace it. Put the motivation and excitement you have now into action. Go to the store and buy some lean protein for dinner right now. Go to the gym and start getting to know the weights right now. Take that first step right now, and you'll build a little momentum that will carry you into more great choices tomorrow.

When motivation courses through your veins and you feel like doing the stuff you just read, you'd damn well better take advantage of it. Otherwise, it's like winning the lottery but not turning in the ticket.

Motivation is finite; it's cyclical. Sometimes you have it, then sometimes it's gone. If you're motivated right now, use it to your advantage to start ingraining these new habits. That way, when motivation wanes, you've built up momentum. You can keep going.

Even in your most motivated moments, it's important to articulate the purpose behind your actions instead of relying on good feelings. When you don't "feel like it," what will keep you going? What is going to sustain you to persevere when motivation vanishes? I've seen people start off excited and feeling great; then things get difficult and they're at a loss. They think, "How do I keep going now?" They neglected to find a purpose to sustain them. The purpose has been discussed at length in this book.

On the flip side, if you've read this far but don't feel particularly motivated, what then? Take action anyway. Action produces results. Quite often, action *precedes* motivation, because action leads to results that can be seen and felt, and they create motivation to keep going, to achieve more.

## LET THE JOURNEY BEGIN

The journey before you is about becoming the best version of yourself. It's my sincerest hope that this book is the catalyst that helps you boldly become more. You're armed with the information you need. If at any point you feel frustrated or confused, look back through the book for guidance.

This is not a journey *to* become more. There's no destination. It's a journey *of* becoming more, in whatever ways you choose. It's a process. A lifestyle. A commitment you renew daily to treat yourself with kindness, compassion, and respect. It's a journey that you approach with excitement and determination to discover your abilities and highlight your strengths.

And it begins now.

# ACKNOWLEDGMENTS

Just as a musician is influenced by the bands and musicians she listened to growing up—they influenced the lyrics she would write, as well as the style in which she played her instrument—so too is a strength coach influenced by other great coaches. I'd like to acknowledge a few of them here.

First, my mom. She is the one who introduced me to strength training, and she blazed the personal-training trail for women in my hometown. It's because of her that I got into fitness and started lifting weights with a determination to discover the amazing things my body could do. I later learned from great instructors and professors at the University of Louisville where I got a bachelor of science in exercise physiology. Thank you, Mom and Doug.

Other great coaches I've learned from who've shared their knowledge in books, articles, seminars, and conversations include Tony Gentilcore, Brad Schoenfeld, Bret Contreras, Mark Rippetoe, Tom Venuto, Dan John, Stuart McRobert, Brooks Kubik, Mike Robertson, Dr. Spencer Nadolsky, Jordan Syatt, Eric Cressey, and Martin Berkhan, and I know there are more. When it comes to nutrition, I have to thank Alan Aragon, Leigh Peele, Georgie Fear, Precision Nutrition, and Examine.com for sharing their knowledge.

Elizabeth, Barbara, Chelsea, and Ellie—this book wouldn't be what it is without you.

## WOULD YOU TAKE A MOMENT TO LEAVE A REVIEW?

Thank you for reading *Lift Like a Girl.*

If you enjoyed this book and found it useful, I'd be honored if you took a few moments to leave a review on Amazon. It will help other women find this book and benefit from it too.

## WANT MORE GREAT INFORMATION?

For a free resource guide with frequently asked questions, additional exercise and nutrition notes, and much more information to help guide you on your *Lift Like a Girl* journey, visit *www.niashanks.com/book-resource-guide/.*

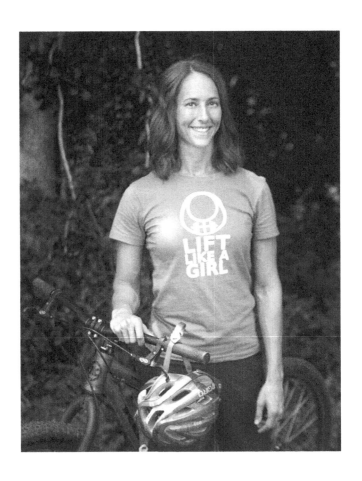

## ABOUT THE AUTHOR

**Nia Shanks** is a fitness coach and writer with a bachelor of science in exercise physiology from the University of Louisville. She specializes in helping women "unleash their awesome" with an empowering approach to health and fitness. Nia's philosophy revolves around strength training programs with a focus on getting stronger and flexible, as well as obsession-free nutrition principles. Through her popular blog and online coaching courses, Nia has helped thousands of women look beyond "quick weight loss" and discover the amazing body they never knew they had.

Made in the USA
Las Vegas, NV
31 October 2022